Task
Analysis

An Individual and Population Approach

Second Edition

Diane E. Watson, PhD, MBA, BScOT
Sylvia A. Wilson, MSc, OT

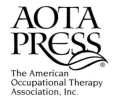

AOTA PRESS

The American
Occupational Therapy
Association, Inc.

Mission Statement

The American Occupational Therapy Association advances the quality, availability, use, and support of occupational therapy through standard-setting, advocacy, education, and research on behalf of its members and the public.

AOTA Staff

Joseph C. Isaacs, CAE, Executive Director
Karen C. Carey, CAE, Associate Executive Director, Membership, Marketing, and Communications

Chris Davis, Managing Editor, AOTA Press
Suzanne Seitz, Production Editor, AOTA Press
Barbara Dickson, Editorial Assistant

Robert A. Sacheli, Manager, Creative Services
Sarah E. Ely, Book Production Coordinator

The American Occupational Therapy Association, Inc.
4720 Montgomery Lane
PO Box 31220
Bethesda, MD 20824-1220
Phone: 301-652-AOTA (2682)
TDD: 800-377-8555
Fax: 301-652-7711
www.aota.org
To order: 1-877-404-AOTA (2682)

Library of Congress Control Number: 2003104338

ISBN: 1-56900-182-0

Disclaimers

This publication is designed to provide accurate and authoritative information in regard to the subject matter covered. It is sold or distributed with the understanding that the publisher is not engaged in rendering legal, accounting, or other professional service. If legal advice or other expert assistance is required, the services of a competent professional person should be sought.
—*From the Declaration of Principles jointly adopted by the American Bar Association and a Committee of Publishers and Associations*

It is the objective of The American Occupational Therapy Association to be a forum for free expression and interchange of ideas. The opinions expressed by the contributors to this work are their own and not necessarily those of The American Occupational Therapy Association.

Design by Sarah E. Ely
Cover by Debra Naylor, Naylor Design
Composition by Maryland Composition Company, Inc., Glen Burnie, MD
Printed by Victor Graphics, Inc., Baltimore, MD

*To my first family, Wayne, Geri, David, Don, and Drew;
my husband Gregg; and my children Austin and Moraya,
who together have encouraged, inspired, and supported me.*

—Diane Watson

*To a family that always joins me in my ventures, Ron,
Kelsey, Nicole, Karlee, and Gregory Wilson, and to my
deceased parents, Paul and Daria Mandziuk, who taught
me to be persistent and tireless when meeting a goal, which
helped tremendously when writing this book.*

—Sylvia Wilson

*The health of the people is really the foundation upon which
all their happiness and all their powers as a state depend.*

—Benjamin Disraeli, July 24, 1877

Contents

List of Tables, Figures, and Case Studies

Foreword

The focus of this book—task analysis—is a foundational skill for occupational therapy practitioners. Identifying the many variables that must be considered when analyzing a task is crucial to effectively being able to select, grade, and adapt activities to help individuals engage in daily life occupations. The authors use a task analysis process and provide a form that includes all of the aspects of the domain outlined in the *Occupational Therapy Practice Framework: Domain and Process* (American Occupational Therapy Association, 2002). This encourages the use of the most current terms and concepts and ensures that learners will attend to all aspects of evaluation. To further encourage learning and integration of these ideas, task analysis cases are presented for individuals across the life span—childhood, adolescence, adulthood, and older adulthood. A wide variety of occupation categories are also addressed. Of particular interest is the chapter on social participation as an occupation. Social participation was the one new category identified in the *Framework* as an area of occupation that had not been previously identified in the *Uniform Terminology III* (which was replaced by the *Framework*).

The publication of *Task Analysis: An Individual and Population Approach, Second Edition* closely intersects with the adoption of the *Framework* and is one of the first texts to incorporate the *Framework's* concepts and language. By choosing to incorporate the *Framework's* ideas and language into their text, the authors have provided practitioners, educators, and students with a vital resource for learning how to apply and use the concepts and language outlined in the *Framework*. The *Framework* is a pivotal document for our profession's thinking. It updates our language to reflect current knowledge and more clearly explicates our domain and process, linking them both firmly to occupation. The fortunate juxtaposition of the publication of this text with the adoption of the *Framework* provides readers with an approach to task analysis that incorporates these new constructs and ideas.

The authors have made a conscious effort to apply task analysis not only to the needs of individuals or small groups but also to populations and communities. The book discusses how task analysis can be used to understand the occupational health and wellness needs of communities and populations. The concrete examples provided will encourage practitioners to enter community practice with increased confidence and provide support for ideas proposed in the *Framework*.

By using the *Framework* as a structure for the process of task analysis the authors have ensured that thinking about task analysis will be grounded in the profession's domain—helping individuals to engage in occupations and to support participation in context. ■

—*Mary Jane Youngstrom, MS, OTR, FAOTA*

Preface

As occupational therapy practitioners, we seek to use meaningful and purposeful activities to create experiences that our clients value. In parallel with this tradition, we wrote *Task Analysis: An Individual and Population Approach* to create a meaningful and purposeful context for learning that we hope our readers will value.

Task analysis is the process of analyzing the dynamic relation among a client, a selected task, and specific contexts—in other words, persons, occupations, and environments. This text focuses on the use of task analysis as a clinical reasoning tool that provides a stepping-stone to the development and refinement of the art and science of occupational performance analysis. Occupational performance analysis focuses on the attainment of a broad understanding of the full range of a client's current and desired occupations, client factors, and performance skills and performance contexts and an appreciation for the complexity of the interactions among these determinants of health. This is the primary clinical reasoning talent of the occupational therapy practitioner.

Task analysis requires consideration of client's performance patterns (i.e., roles, habits, and routines), performance skills (i.e., process, motor, communication, and interaction), client factors (i.e., body structures and functions), activity demands, and contextual factors (i.e., environmental and personal). We derived this framework for structuring the analysis from the *Occupational Therapy Practice Framework: Domain and Process* (American Occupational Therapy Association [AOTA], 2002), which outlines the terminology we use in this volume.

Analysis of the demands inherent in engagement in purposeful activities has historically been called *activity analysis* by occupational therapy practitioners, but it is only one step in the process of conducting task analysis; it is the part that focuses on an activity or occupation. The purpose of activity analysis is to determine whether an activity has restorative potential or value and how to grade therapeutic activities (Moyers, 1999; Watson, 1997). In keeping with Llorens (1993) and others (e.g., Cynkin, 1979; Mosey, 1986; Trombly, 1995a), this text uses the term *activity analysis* to refer to the skill of analyzing an activity or process to determine whether it motivates and fulfills a client's needs and whether it enhances client factors, performance skills, and personal factors. Because task analysis requires an assessment of the activity demands of a selected task, we see activity analysis as a subset of task analysis.

We elected to use the problem-based approach to learning because we believe it creates a realistic and rewarding context for developing clinical reasoning. The people and circumstances in these case profiles are hypothetical (with the exception of the case study of CATCH in chapter 17) and are intended to provide meaningful contexts for learning; any similarity to real persons or events is purely coincidental. Although the cases in this book are hypothetical, the issues are representational. Problem-based learning should refine readers' skills in narrative, interactive, procedural, and conditional clinical reasoning (Van Leit, 1995). The realism of the case profiles will enable readers to practice the cognitive steps and professional behaviors required of knowledgeable and skilled practitioners. The learning experiences are developmental and integrative, and challenge questions at the end of each chapter provide ample opportunity for readers to determine the focus of their learning experience. The problem-based approach to learning complements the occupational therapy profession's belief that meaningful engagement sanctions diversity and flexibility in learning and adaptation (Watson, 1997). It parallels the profession's tradition of using purposeful activity to promote learning, insight, skills, and independent and self-directed performance.

In occupational therapy the term *client* has evolved to include any entity that receives services. Clients may be individuals (e.g., patient, student, teacher, caregiver), individuals in the context of a group (e.g., family, students), or individuals within the context of a population (i.e., a community) (AOTA, 2002). Our book also includes the community collective as an entity. Although the most common form of service delivery in the late 1990s and early 2000s is directed toward individual clients, more and more practitioners serve clients at the group and population level and are involved in community development initiatives. Because many people in our profession do not have experience applying task analysis to populations, we designed this text for use by occupational therapy students, educators, and practitioners.

The first edition of this book, *Task Analysis: An Occupational Performance Approach,* originally included a section on how to use task analysis to guide services to individuals and communities (Watson, 1997). Since that time our understanding of this emerging area of practice has been enriched by the work of several scholars and practitioners who work in the areas of community development, public health, and population health. This enriched understanding led us to the framework we propose for the application of task analysis to populations (chapter 15). The merits of the model we propose have not been confirmed by research; we simply offer our professional experience in applying task analysis to promote healthy communities. Over the past decade, one of the authors of this text (Wilson) has worked closely with communities to promote health in their customary contexts. The other (Watson) has worked closely with the health services research and policy community to ground public policy and health care services in evidence to promote the health of populations. In both contexts, we use task analysis to understand the dynamic interaction between persons and their occupations and contexts and to design interventions that promote health. We hope our approach to applying task analysis to populations is used, evaluated, and further developed by occupational therapy practitioners who seek to work in this emerging service arena.

One occupational therapy scholar defined an *occupation* as a "specific individual's personally constructed, non-repeatable experience . . . a subjective event in perceived temporal, spatial, and sociocultural conditions that are unique to that one-time occurrence" (Pierce, 2001, 139). The process of writing this book has been a meaningful occupation for both of us; we hope that reading it will be a purposeful occupation for you! ■

Acknowledgments

A few key people have heavily influenced the occupation of writing this book, and the contexts in which we have lived our lives laid the foundation on which this book was written. We address the former and the latter together, as people and contexts are inseparable in their influence on our lives.

Although many people at the Department of Occupational Therapy at the University of Alberta introduced us to the profession, Sharon Brintnell and Helen Madill in particular have continued to enrich our understanding over the past 20 to 30 years. Through chance meetings and occasional dinners, they have enlightened our understanding of the history, applicability, and potential of the profession and its beliefs. We also credit the many people involved in the creation of the person–environment–occupation model of occupational performance (Law et al., 1996). They must be congratulated for "simplifying the recipe." Many other scholars have influenced this work, and they are cited in the reference list.

The first edition of *Task Analysis* acknowledged 30 different people for their valued contribution to that text. As this work builds on theirs, we continue to owe credit. The first edition was created out of a collaborative effort between one author, Diane Watson, and the occupational therapy graduating class of 1998 from the University of Scranton in Pennsylvania. These practitioners, and Dr. Jack Kasar, who was the department chair at the time, each contributed to the success of the first edition and have laid the foundation we used to create the second edition. Occupations as intense and all-consuming as writing a book also require supportive performance contexts at work and home. Our husbands (Ron and Gregg) and our children (Kelsey, Nicole, Karlee, Gregory, Austin, and Moraya) missed us, and it is to their needs that we now turn our attention.

Many experts in various areas of specialty have reviewed versions of this manuscript, and their formative feedback has influenced the contents of these pages. We are particularly grateful for the extensive comments and feedback of anonymous reviewers. Gregg Landry was very helpful in framing the breadth and scope of this second edition and ensuring its timely completion. The editors and staff at the American Occupational Therapy Association also contributed substantially to the quality and timely completion of this project.

We owe tremendous gratitude to Nicole

Wilson and Geri Watson. Nicole applied her talents at photography to take all of the pictures in this text. As you can see for yourself, without these images the book would not focus so much attention on the importance of engaging in occupations and participating in contexts. Geri was our editor-in-chief during the manuscript preparation phase. She had the courage to criticize and knew when to be gentle. Between Geri and the authors, we have 95 years of experience as occupational therapy practitioners in diverse practice environments across Canada and the United States. It would be impossible to count the clients we have collectively served, but it is they who have taught us the art of applying task analysis to occupational therapy practice. ▪

I

Introduction

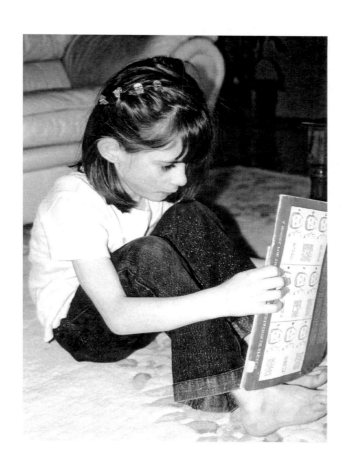

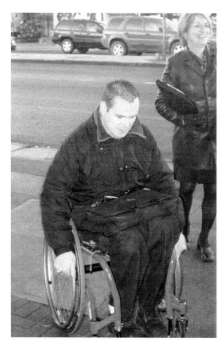

CHAPTER 1

Occupational Therapy Services: Contributing to Health and Wellness

Occupational therapy practitioners apply their art and science to direct a client's involvement in selected tasks, and it is the sum of these engagements in tasks that becomes engagement in occupations and participation in contexts. Task analysis is a clinical reasoning tool practitioners use to analyze occupational performance and design interventions targeted at people, environments, and/or occupations.

CHAPTER OBJECTIVES
- To describe occupational therapy's contribution to health and wellness.
- To describe the profession's focus on engagement in occupations and participation in contexts.

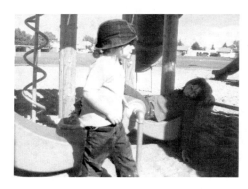

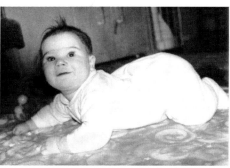

Occupational Therapy Services: Contributing to Health and Wellness

O ccupational therapy has a long tradition of helping clients improve their health and wellness. This tradition has been shaped over generations by its practitioners' enduring commitment to promote their clients' engagement in occupations and participation in contexts. This chapter frames occupational therapy's contribution to health and wellness by describing its key concepts, including *evaluation and intervention services, engagement in occupation to support participation,* and *health and wellness.* These elements form a logic chain that starts with services and ends with health and wellness, as illustrated in Figure 1.1.

How does one define what it is like to experience health and wellness? The American Occupational Therapy Association (AOTA, 2002) uses the World Health Organization's (WHO, 1948) definition of *health:* "a complete state of physical, mental, and social well-being and not just the absence of disease and infirmity" (p. 100). AOTA (2002) has defined *wellness* as both a condition of being in good health, including appreciating and enjoying that health, and a state of mental and physical balance and fitness. WHO is the United Nations' specialized agency for health, and as such it has produced guidelines

to provide a unifying and standard language and framework to understand, describe, and study health, health-related states, outcomes, and determinants (WHO, 2001).

What contributes to a person's or population's health and well-being? Broad constructs of health and well-being include the following conditions and resources as fundamental determinants of health: peace, shelter, education, food, income, a stable ecosystem, sustainable resources, social justice, and equity (WHO, 1986). The components of health and health-related states include body functions and structures, engagement in activities and participation in life situations, and environmental factors (WHO, 2001).

Occupational Therapy Concepts

Occupational therapy offers a distinct approach to the promotion of health and wellness; the profession provides services that enable clients to engage in occupations to support participation in their contexts. WHO (2001) defined *participation* as "involvement in a life situation" (p. 10), and Law (2002a) defined it as "involvement in formal and informal everyday activities" (p. 641).

In 2002 the AOTA published *Occupational Therapy Practice Framework: Domain and Process,*

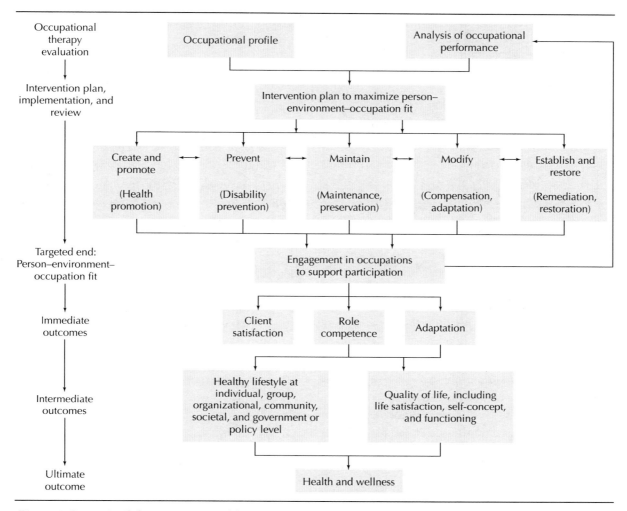

Figure 1.1. Occupational therapy services model.

which established *engagement in occupation to support participation* as the profession's targeted end. The *Framework* described in this document articulates the profession's current thinking on the domain and process of the profession, and occupational therapy practitioners must be familiar with its contents. Youngstrom (2002), a participant in the AOTA Commission on Practice, explained the Commission's choices of terms used in the *Framework* as follows:

> The phrase "engagement in occupation to support participation" was purposefully chosen to point out several key ideas that describe the profession's understanding of occupation and its contribution to health. The term "engagement" was chosen because it depicts

the personal commitment and meaning that are associated with carrying out occupations. Engagement implies that the performance of occupations includes psychological and emotional elements as well as physical actions. The words "to support participation" were purposefully placed after "engagement in occupation" to illustrate that occupational therapists believe that supporting individuals to engage in occupations allows them to naturally make the transition to participation in a variety of real-life contexts that are meaningful to them.... Positioning occupational therapy in this domain makes a clear statement about occupational therapy's contribution to health—a focus on helping clients (individuals, groups, or organizations) to engage in occupations (i.e., daily life activities that are purposeful, meaningful and important to the client) that enable their participation in life situations. (p. 608)

The prevalence of chronic impairments, activity limitations, and participation restrictions is increasing in the population as a whole (McNeil, 1993, 1997; U.S. Department of Health and Human Services, 2001). Changes in the nature and distribution of health and illness risks, coupled with an enhanced understanding of the determinants of health and illness, have led occupational therapy practitioners to offer services not only to individual clients who seek to improve their engagement and participation but also to communities and populations of people who are committed to promoting the health and well-being of their members. Whether with individuals or groups, occupational therapy practitioners target their evaluation and intervention to optimize the interactions among people, their environments, and their occupations. For it is this interaction that contributes to people's engagement in occupations and participation in contexts and, ultimately, to the health of individuals and populations.

Occupational therapy practice is a *client-centered service* in that practitioners collaborate with clients and their proxies and focus priorities on the issues their clients identify. The term *client* refers to the entity that receives services, and clients may be individuals (e.g., patient, student, teacher, caregiver, lawyer), individuals in the context of a group (e.g., family, students), or individuals within the context of a population (e.g., agencies, governments, corporations) (AOTA, 2002; Law, Polatajko, Baptiste, & Townsend, 1997). Populations can be defined on the basis of geography (e.g., local community) or of shared characteristics (e.g., children, students, older adults, persons with disabilities). All of these clientele may benefit from occupational therapy. Often other professionals also work with occupational therapy clients, and clients are best served when their occupational therapy practitioners establish partnerships and work in collaboration with such professionals in areas of mutual interest.

Occupational therapy practitioners have traditionally worked with clients who have or who are at risk for disabilities. *Disability* is an umbrella term for impairments, activity limitations, and participation restrictions (WHO, 2001). *Impairments* are problems in body function (i.e., physiology) and structure (i.e., anatomy) that result in significant deviation or loss in that which is considered normal functions or structures. *Activity limitations* are difficulties in executing a task, and *participation restrictions* are problems experienced in involvement in life situations. The term *involvement* means "taking part, being included or engaged in an area of life, being accepted, or having access to needed resources," and it can be gauged through performance (WHO, 2001, p. 13). WHO's focus on engagement and on participation is echoed in the definition of the targeted outcome of occupational therapy provided in the *Occupational Therapy Practice Framework* (AOTA, 2002).

Occupational therapy services begin with *evaluation,* during which the occupational therapist focuses on the establishment of an occupational profile of the client and an analysis of his or her occupational performance. Evaluation enables the occupational therapist to understand the client and his or her environments and occupations and to design an intervention to optimize the fit among these areas of concern. Developing an occupational profile, analyzing occupational performance, and using this information to plan and review intervention require a broad understanding of the client and his or her current and desired occupations, activity demands, and performance contexts, and an appreciation for the complexity of the interactions among these dimensions (AOTA, 2002). Occupational therapy practitioners apply their art and science in using this information to direct a client's involvement in selected tasks, and it is the sum of these engagements in tasks that becomes engagement in occupations and participation in contexts. Task analysis, which is discussed in more detail in chapter 4, is thus a key component of occupational therapy evaluation. *Task analysis* is the process of analyzing the dynamic interaction among a client, his or her environments, and selected tasks (a subset of occupation) and designing intervention to optimize the fit among these three dimensions.

Theories, approaches, models of practice, and frames of reference guide occupational therapy evaluation and intervention. This text does not focus on theories but provides ample opportunity for readers to apply their theoretical knowledge to the case studies in the following chapters. As illustrated in Figure 1.1, occupational therapy practitioners choose from among several *approaches* to intervention, including health promotion, disability prevention, maintenance, compensation or adaptation, and remediation or restoration. They may use different types of interventions within each of these approaches, and although "engagement in occupations to support participation" is the targeted end of service delivery, other service outcomes of interventions are expected. Appendixes G and H describe and define approaches to and types of intervention, and Appendix I lists expected outcomes of intervention.

The focus of this text is on teaching a model of practice and its application through task analysis when services are directed toward individuals and populations. *Models of practice* provide a guide to day-to-day practice and to how occupational therapy practitioners think about what they do as health professionals. Models help one to understand complex relations among concepts and components and determine what professionals consider important to their reasoning about clients (Canadian Association of Occupational Therapists, 2002). The person–environment–occupation (PEO) model of occupational performance, discussed in chapter 2, describes what occupational therapy practitioners think about in their day-to-day practice when they seek to promote engagement in occupations and participation in contexts (Law et al., 1996).

Frames of reference provide structure to help people organize and apply knowledge. The frame of reference we use in this book consists of the domain (engagement in occupation to support participation in contexts) and dimensions (areas of occupation, performance skills, performance patterns, contexts, activity demands, and client factors; see Appendixes A through F) of occupational therapy practice defined in the *Occupational Therapy Practice Framework* (AOTA, 2002).

A historical perspective on occupational performance and task analysis is provided in chapter 2. The domains and dimensions are discussed in more detail in chapter 3, and chapter 4 describes the process of practice. Chapters 5 and 15 discuss the similarities and differences in the occupational therapy process when services are directed toward individuals and populations. Chapter 6 illustrates the range of occupations people engage in throughout their lives. Client case studies in chapters 7–14 focus primarily on services to individuals, and client case studies in chapters 16–18 focus on services to populations.

The Challenge

1. Reflect on Youngstrom's (2002) description of the AOTA Commission on Practice's rationale for defining the targeted outcome of the occupational therapy process as "engagement in occupation to support participation." Then reflect on the definitions of participation proposed by WHO (2001) and Law (2002a). From your personal perspective, how do engagement in occupations and participation in contexts have a positive effect on you and others?

2. Read the Distinguished Scholar Lecture entitled "Participation in Occupations of Everyday Life" by Law (2002a). Describe the nature of participation, and reflect on your own experiences regarding participation in occupations. Then describe the influence of participation on health and well-being.

3. Reflect on your personal experience, values, and beliefs about health and wellness to better understand WHO and AOTA definitions of these important concepts. What is it like to feel healthy and experience well-being? Describe

what "state of health and well-being" means to you.

Identify and list things that contribute to a state of health. Cluster these items into one or more of the following three categories: person, environment, and occupation. For example, if you describe health and well-being as including a sense of personal security and identify public safety as a determinant of this state of health, then write *sense of security* in the person category and *safe public places* in the environment category.

4. Write a short list of tasks and their component activities that are important to you in one or more of the following areas of occupation: activities of daily living, education, work, play, leisure, and social participation. Consider the

types of questions you might ask to obtain this type of information from a client. The following are examples: "What is it that you enjoy doing most?" "How did your interest develop?" "What level of satisfaction do you get from accomplishing the task or activity?"

Practice interviewing another person to determine what occupations, tasks, and activities are important to him or her. Use the information you collect from your interviewee to draft an occupational profile that identifies his or her interests, values, beliefs, and needs. As you work through the chapters of this book, you will learn step by step how to enrich this profile through a more thorough analysis of a client's contexts, activity demands, and performance skills and patterns. ▪

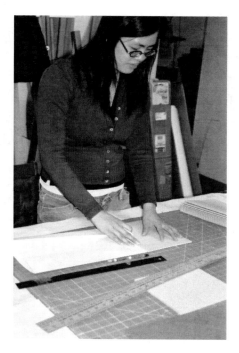

CHAPTER 2

Historical Perspectives on Activities, Occupations, and Participation

Engagement in occupation to support participation in context is the focus and targeted end objective of occupational therapy intervention.

—American Occupational Therapy Association, 2002, p. 611

CHAPTER OBJECTIVES

■ To define the terms *purposeful activity, occupation,* and *occupational performance.*

■ To explain and illustrate the concept of *fit* among persons, environments, and occupations.

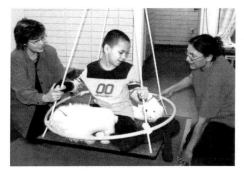

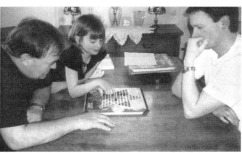

Historical Perspectives on Activities, Occupations, and Participation

The belief that engagement in activity has healing power has its roots in the Arts and Crafts movement of the late 19th century and in the philosophies of the founders of occupational therapy. Early occupational therapy theorists acknowledged the unity among mind, body, and spirit and the linkage among engagement, self-fulfillment, and health (Atwood, 1907; Meyer, 1922; Moher, 1907). Goal-directed activities to instill craftsmanship and workplace skills were used as diversions as well as for therapeutic, vocational, and motivational benefit.

Evolving Focus of the Profession

Terms used to describe early occupational therapy included *work treatment, work therapy, occupational re-education,* and *work cure* (Hall, 1910; Hopkins, 1988). The term *occupational therapy* was apparently coined by George Barton, who saw therapists as curing patients through the use of work (Dunlop, 1933). Barton was an architect who experienced disabling conditions that led him to pursue studies in the field of rehabilitation. Through these pursuits he made contact with the contemporary leaders of the field—Dr. William R. Dutton, Eleanor Clark Slagle, Susan Tracey,

and Susan Cox Johnson (Sabonis-Chafee & Hussey, 1998). As Polatajko (2001) observed,

> Our evolution started with a concept of occupation that was akin to the present day concept of work, not necessarily paid work, but work none the less.... It was considered that the absence of work, in and of itself, resulted in the deterioration of the human condition and that the only remedy was work. (p. 204)

Other early theorists saw the potential domain of occupational therapy as much broader and more health related than vocational training (Friedland, 2001; Kidner, 1923). The following definition of *occupational therapy* was proposed in 1921: "any activity, mental or physical, definitely prescribed and guided for the distinct purpose of contributing to and hastening recovery from disease or injury" (Hall, 1922, p. 61). This broader conceptualization of the domain of occupational therapy soon dominated the field; although early scholars wrote about the concept of occupation until the 1930s, the only consistent use of the term *occupation* between the 1940s and 1980s was in the title of the profession. The profession's literature during that period focused around the term *activity* and the therapeutic use of activity.

During the 1960s and 1970s, occupational therapy leaders advocated a focus not only on returning patients to previous activities but also on helping people engage in meaningful occupations and participate in life (Polatajko, 2001). By 2002 the focus on participation was ratified in the official definition of the domain of the profession: "engagement in occupation to support participation in context or contexts" (American Occupational Therapy Association [AOTA], 2002, p. 611). "Participation is the raison d'être of occupational therapy; it is what we are all about; it is our unique contribution to society" (Law, 2002a, p. 640).

Activities

Activity analysis has been used as an approach to determining whether an activity is meaningful, motivates and fulfills a client's needs, and can be used to help him or her attain the therapeutic aims of developing or restoring skills and abilities. Activity analysis enables occupational therapy practitioners to determine whether an activity has therapeutic potential or value and to select and design an activity to treat a disability or functional limitation (Trombly, 1995a). The purpose of activity analysis is to determine whether an activity has restorative potential or value and to grade therapeutic activities (Watson, 1997).

Occupational therapy practitioners and educators incorporated activity analysis into practice and educational programs during World War I (Creighton, 1992). Joint position, action, and muscle strength were of primary interest, as was analysis of the abilities required to engage in a specific activity. By the 1920s, Haas (1922) suggested a system of activity analysis and rating. Activities were classified according to their therapeutic benefits between 1920 and the 1940s, and through the 1960s, analyses included physical requirements and emotional and social properties. Then, during the 1970s, 1980s, and 1990s, several frames of reference influenced activity analysis methods, requiring practitioners to recognize sensorimotor, affective, cognitive, biomechanical, volitional,

contextual, and spiritual parameters (Canadian Association of Occupational Therapy [CAOT], 1997; Creighton, 1992).

Throughout the 20th century, occupational therapy practitioners developed their skills in activity analysis to select and design therapeutic activities as modalities for use in attaining client goals. Early in the century, Gilbreth (1911) introduced the concept of job analysis through motion studies. Motion studies involved analysis of characteristics of the worker, the worker's surroundings, and the motion requirements of the job, and these studies enabled practitioners to recommend adaptations to improve efficiency. Friedman (1916) recommended that health professionals seeking to match clients with a vocation consider the physical, mental, and psychological requirements of the particular occupation. Thus, occupational therapy leaders have historically recognized the significance of a fit among persons, environments, and occupations, and this tenet continues to dominate the profession to this day.

By analyzing the features, characteristics, and qualities of activities, occupational therapy practitioners realized that they could grade and modify activities and tasks according to the client's residual capabilities and prescribe purposeful activities as therapeutic modalities (Hinojosa, Sabari, & Rosenfeld, 1983; Kidner, 1930). Activities are deemed to be purposeful when they (a) are relevant, meaningful, and goal directed; (b) elicit coordination among sensorimotor, cognitive, psychological, and psychosocial systems; and (c) promote mastery and feelings of competence (AOTA, 1993; Fidler & Fidler, 1978; Trombly, 1995b).

Occupations

Occupations are activities that have meaning and purpose in a person's life; they are central to identity and competence and influence how one spends time and makes decisions (AOTA, 2002).

> Occupational therapists and occupational therapy assistants focus on assisting people to engage in daily life activities that they find meaningful and purposeful.... The term that

occupational therapists and occupational therapy assistants use to capture the breadth and meaning of "everyday life activity" is occupation. (AOTA, 2002, p. 610)

The experience of engaging in an occupation generally has a distinct, subjective meaning for each individual. For example, "those who experience gardening as an occupation would see themselves as gardeners, gaining part of their identity from their participation" (AOTA, 2002, p. 610). By engaging clients' minds, spirits, and bodies in occupations, occupational therapy practitioners facilitate optimal engagement and participation. This approach distinguishes occupational therapy from verbal therapy (CAOT, 1993).

Participation

By the early 1990s and through to the present, the profession has incorporated participation as a tenet (AOTA, 2002; CAOT, 1997, Polatajko, 1992). Definitions of the profession place a strong value on the occupational therapy practitioner's role in supporting participation in contexts through engagement in occupations:

> Occupational therapy is the art and science of directing an individual's participation in selected tasks to restore, reinforce, and enhance performance; facilitate learning of those skills and functions essential for adaptation and productivity; diminish or correct pathology; and promote and maintain health. (AOTA, 1995a, p. 89; AOTA, 1995b, p. 105)

Law (2002a), reflecting on the importance of participation, observed the following:

> Participation in the everyday occupations of life is a vital part of human development and lived experience. Through participation we acquire skills and competencies, connect with others and our communities, and find meaning and purpose in life. As members of the profession of occupational therapy, we seek to improve health and well-being through occupation. Occupational therapy focuses on enabling individuals and groups to participate in everyday occupations that are meaningful to them, provide fulfillment, and engage them in everyday life with others. Our focus is on enhancing participation. (p. 640)

Occupational Performance: The Person–Environment–Occupation Model

In the early 1970s, AOTA proposed that the role, function, and domain of concern of occupational therapy practitioners were occupational performance (AOTA, 1973, 1974). *Occupational performance* is the accomplishment of a selected occupation, task, or activity resulting from the dynamic interaction among clients, their environments, and their occupations (AOTA, 1994a). In response to regulatory requirements for uniform reporting systems, a national uniform terminology system was first developed and approved in 1979. This document started to frame the profession's view of the determinants of occupational performance and the domain of concern to the profession (AOTA, 1979). Its third edition, *Uniform Terminology for Occupational Therapy* (AOTA, 1994a), proposed that practice focus on three domains: performance areas, performance components, and performance contexts. At that time, optimal occupational performance was deemed to occur when there was a fit, or match, among persons, activities, and environments that resulted in enhanced participation. The purpose of intervention was seen as the creation of a fit among the person, the activity, and the environment by aligning "the skills and abilities of the individual; the demands of activity; and the characteristics of the physical, social, and cultural environments" (AOTA, 1994a, p. 277).

As part of the review process to update and revise *Uniform Terminology for Occupational Therapy,* the AOTA Commission on Practice again updated the profession's domain of concern (AOTA, 2002). The new *Framework* adheres to the concept of interaction and fit among person, environment, and occupation.

> Execution of a performance skill occurs when the performer, the context, and the demands of the activity come together in the performance of the activity. Each of these factors influences the execution of a skill and may support or hinder actual skill execution. (AOTA, 2002, p. 612)

An occupational performance approach to evaluation and intervention focuses on the dynamic, interdependent, and transactional relations among persons (i.e., clients), environments (i.e., contexts), and occupations (Law, et al., 1996; 2002). The person–environment–occupation (PEO) model holds that occupational performance is shaped by the continuous and simultaneous interaction among these dimensions (CAOT, 1993; Law, 2002a; Law et al., 1996; Law, Polatajko, Baptiste, & Townsend, 1997). Figure 2.1 depicts the three dimensions of the PEO with occupational performance represented in the overlap of the dimension. This model, which provides a holistic perspective on the domain of occupational therapy, increases the scope of assessment options and intervention strategies available to practitioners beyond activity analysis (Dunn, Brown, & McGuigan, 1994; Law et al., 1996; Letts et al., 1994).

The PEO model of occupational performance clarifies the conceptualization of fit by focusing attention on the interaction among, and overlap of, dimensions in the model. As depicted in Figure 2.2, separate but interconnected spheres represent the person, the environment, and the occupation. Overlap among the spheres represents occupational performance. Optimal occupational performance occurs when the overlap among the spheres is maximized and the person, environment, and occupation appear inseparable (Figure 2.2). When the interaction of the three dimensions of the model is harmonious or compatible, occupational performance is optimal, as is a client's engagement in occupations and participation in contexts. As depicted in Figure 2.3, the interactions among the dimensions vary across time and are reflected in the changing performance patterns (i.e., habits, roles, and routines) of persons (Law et al., 1996). The factors that contribute to temporal changes in the interactions are those conditions or situations that contribute to or influence health.

The Challenge

1. Define the terms *purposeful activity, occupation,* and *occupational performance.*
2. Occupations have been described as "chunks" of tasks and activities that occur within the context of culture (Frank, 1996b). Describe the cultural context in which the task of fishing is seen as a work occupation, and describe the cultural context in which fishing is seen as a leisure occupation. How are the meaning and purpose of a task or occupation influenced by context?
3. List the array of activities nested in the task of fishing as a work occupation and as a leisure occupation. How do the activities differ between these two occupations? How are the basic needs of people met through fishing as work versus fishing as leisure occupation? In answering the latter question, consider the four functions of occupations identified by Wilcock (1998, p. 89): (a) to provide for immediate bodily needs of sustenance, self-care, and shelter; (b) to develop skills, social structures, and technology aimed at safety and superiority over predators and the environment; (c) to maintain

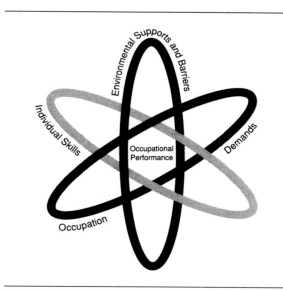

Figure 2.1. PEO model of occupational performance.
From "The Person–Environment–Occupation Model: A Transactive Approach to Occupational Performance" by M. Law, B. Cooper, S. Strong, D. Steward, P. Rigby, & L. Letts, 1996, *Canadian Journal of Occupational Therapy, 63,* 9–23. Copyright 1996 by the Canadian Association of Occupational Therapists (CAOT). Reproduced with permission of CAOT Publications.

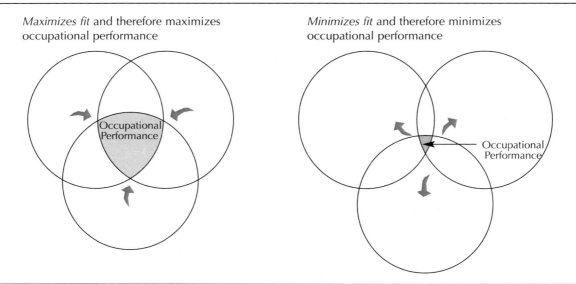

Maximizes *fit* and therefore maximizes
occupational performance

Minimizes *fit* and therefore minimizes
occupational performance

Figure 2.2. An illustration of changes to occupational performance as a consequence of variations in fit among person, environment, and occupation.
From "The Person–Environment–Occupation Model: A Transactive Approach to Occupational Performance" by M. Law, B. Cooper, S. Strong, D. Steward, P. Rigby, & L. Letts, 1996, *Canadian Journal of Occupational Therapy, 63,* 9–23. Copyright 1996 by the Canadian Association of Occupational Therapists (CAOT). Reproduced with permission of CAOT Publications.

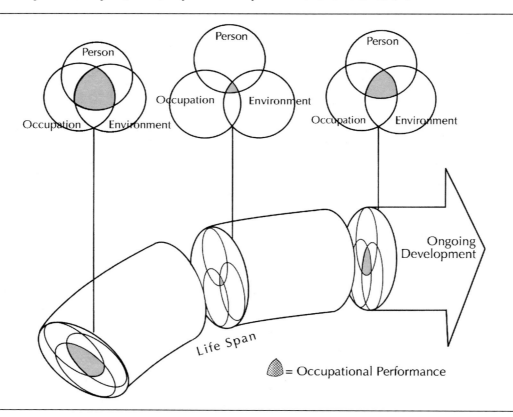

Figure 2.3. Depiction of the person–environment–occupation model of occupational performance across the life span.
From "The Person–Environment–Occupation Model: A Transactive Approach to Occupational Performance" by M. Law, B. Cooper, S. Strong, D. Steward, P. Rigby, & L. Letts, 1996, *Canadian Journal of Occupational Therapy, 63,* 9–23. Copyright 1996 by the Canadian Association of Occupational Therapists (CAOT). Reproduced with permission of CAOT Publications.

health by balanced exercise and personal capacities; and (d) to enable individual and social development so that each person and species will flourish.

4. Select one activity required in the task of fishing as a work or leisure occupation. What are the demands of this activity (i.e., required actions, body functions, and body structures)? Refer to Appendix E for a list of ways to describe the features of activities and the demands they place on clients.

5. Describe the differences among *task analysis, activity analysis,* and *occupational performance analysis.* ▄

Domain and Process of Occupational Therapy

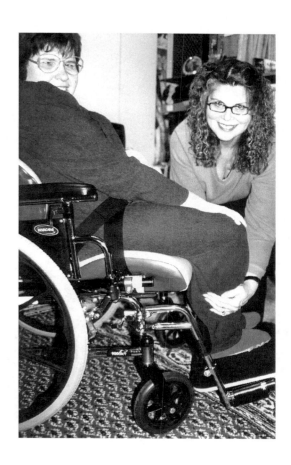

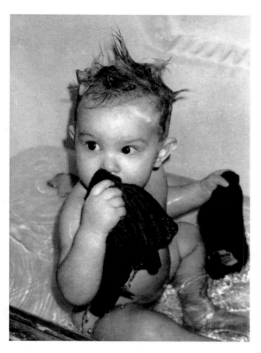

CHAPTER 3

Domain and Dimensions of Occupational Therapy

Occupations are the "activities . . . of everyday life, named, organized, and given value and meaning by individuals and a culture."

—Law, Cooper, Strong, Steward, Rigby, & Letts, 1997, p. 32

CHAPTER OBJECTIVES
- To define the domain and dimensions of concern to occupational therapy practitioners.
- To define *occupation* and *areas of occupation*.
- To identify and define the types of performance skills and patterns, contexts, activity demands, and client factors that influence engagement and participation.

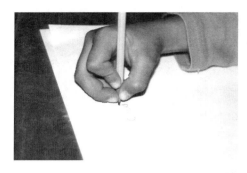

Domain and Dimensions of Occupational Therapy

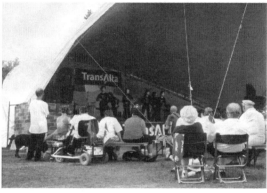

In the late 1990s, the Commission on Practice of the American Occupational Therapy Association (AOTA) undertook a review and consultation process to develop a framework for practice that defines and communicates the domain of the profession and the process of service delivery. The *Occupational Therapy Practice Framework: Domain and Process* (AOTA, 2002) describes the domain of concern to the profession and builds on a historic AOTA document that established a uniform terminology for occupational therapy (AOTA, 1994b). The *Framework* now incorporates terminology from the *International Classification of Functioning, Disability, and Health* (ICF) developed by the World Health Organization (WHO, 2001). This international classification system provides a unified and standard framework for describing health and health-related status, fostering better communication among health practitioners nationally and internationally. This chapter describes occupational therapy's domain of practice and defines the dimensions of this domain as outlined in the *Framework*.

In the *Occupational Therapy Practice Framework*, "the phrase 'engagement in occupation to support participation in context or contexts' was delineated as the overarching theme that describes the profession's domain" (Youngstrom, 2002, p. 608). The domain of the occupational therapy profession has been further defined as "assisting people to engage in daily life activities that they find meaningful and purposeful" (AOTA, 2002, p. 610). This domain provides the foundation on which practitioners construct their activities (Law, 2002a). The occupational therapy service delivery process includes evaluation and intervention that support "engagement in meaningful occupations that subsequently affect health, well-being, and life satisfaction" (AOTA, 2002, p. 610).

Engagement in meaningful occupations is the central focus of occupational therapy. Occupations are the "ordinary and familiar things that people do every day" (Clark et al., 1991, p. 300). Occupations are intrinsically necessary for health and well-being, and engagement in occupations and participation in contexts are driven by the need for mastery, competence, self-identity, and group acceptance (Law et al., 1996; Polatajko, 1994). The complexities lie in the fact that people and their environments and occupations are indivisible. Although occupation is a complex construct, it is a concept people readily understand because everyone engages in it in their daily lives.

The term that occupational therapy practitioners use to capture the breadth and meaning of "everyday life activity" is *occupation:*

> Occupation refers to groups of activities and tasks of everyday life, named, organized, and given value and meaning by individuals and a culture. Occupation is everything people do to occupy themselves, including looking after themselves (self-care), enjoying life (leisure), and contributing to the social and economic fabric of their communities (productivity). (Law, Polatajko, Baptiste, & Townsend, 1997, p. 32)

The profession views the client's engagement in occupation as an end in itself (i.e., an outcome of service) and as a means to an end (i.e., a process of intervention). The targeted end of the intervention process occurs when the client attains maximum engagement in occupations and participation in contexts. By comparison, the service delivery process involves the therapeutic use of purposeful activity and involvement in daily life activities as a means or method of changing levels of engagement and participation. Occupational therapy practitioners contribute to their clients' health by enabling them to choose and engage in occupations that give their lives meaning and purpose (Canadian Association of Occupational Therapists [CAOT], 1993, 1997). Part of the "science" of occupational therapy is to "generate knowledge about the form, the function, and the meaning of human occupation" (Zemke & Clark, 1996, p. vii).

Figure 3.1 lists the dimensions of the domain of occupational therapy as defined by AOTA (2002), and Figure 3.2 overlays these dimensions onto the person–environment–occupation (PEO) model of occupational performance (Law et al., 1996). The domain and its dimensions frame the focus of practitioners' attention during the evaluation and intervention process—namely, the interaction of persons, environments, and occupations. It is the extent and quality of this interaction that determine levels of engagement and participation. The top center circle in Figure 3.2 represents the person and lists the dimensions that influence the

person's engagement in occupations and participation in contexts—namely, personal and spiritual contexts, performance skills and patterns, and body functions and structures. The bottom left circle represents occupation and includes the dimensions of areas of occupation as well as two types of activity demands: objects used and sequencing and timing. The bottom right circle represents environment and includes the physical, social, temporal, and virtual contexts.

The dimensions listed in which person and occupation overlap are the activity demands of required actions and required body structures and functions. Likewise, person and environment overlap in the dimension of cultural context, and occupation and environment overlap in the dimensions of social and space activity demands. The domain of occupational therapy, engagement in occupation, and participation in context requires and is influenced by all of these dimensions. Therefore, this domain is represented in the overlap areas of these dimensions.

No one dimension of the domain of practice is considered more important than another (AOTA, 2002). Appendixes A through F list and define all of the dimensions of the occupational therapy domain.

Occupational therapists are trained to evaluate the interaction of persons, environments, and occupations using task analysis and to apply the knowledge they gain through this analysis to planning and reviewing interventions to facilitate their clients' engagement in occupations and participation in contexts. Occupational therapy assistants participate in this process under the supervision of an occupational therapist.

Areas of Occupation

When occupational therapy practitioners work with an individual, group, community, or population to promote engagement and participation, they take into account all of the areas of occupation identified in Figure 3.1: activities of daily living (ADL), instrumental activities of daily living (IADL), education, work, play, leisure, and social participation. Each of these areas includes several tasks and activities, and a single task or activity may apply to more than one area of occupation.

The ADL area of occupation includes basic and personal activities a person engages in for the purpose of taking care of his or her own body, such as bathing and showering, bowel and bladder management, dressing, eating and feeding, functional mobility, personal device care, hygiene and grooming, sexual activity, sleep and rest, and toilet hygiene. The IADL area of occupation includes tasks required for effective interaction with the environment, such as community mobility, financial management, health maintenance

and management, home maintenance and management, meal preparation and cleanup, safety procedures and emergency responses, and shopping. IADL also include more complex tasks such as caring for others (e.g., children, pets; AOTA, 2002; Rogers & Holm, 1994).

The education area of occupation includes engagement in student roles, participation in learning environments, and formal educational preparation (i.e., academic and extracurricular) as well as exploration and participation in informal personal education. Work occupations are tasks done for remuneration or volunteer purposes and entail the identification and selection of vocational

---

ENGAGEMENT IN OCCUPATION TO SUPPORT PARTICIPATION IN CONTEXT OR CONTEXTS

▨ Performance in Areas of Occupation

Activities of Daily Living (ADL)*
Instrumental Activities of Daily Living (IADL)
Education
Work
Play
Leisure
Social Participation
(For definitions, refer to Appendix A)

▨ Performance Skills	▨ Performance Patterns
Motor Skills	Habits
Process Skills	Routines
Communication/Interaction Skills	Roles
(For definitions, refer to Appendix B)	*(For definitions, refer to Appendix C)*

▨ Context	▨ Activity Demands	▨ Client Factors
Cultural	Objects Used and Their Properties	Body Functions
Physical	Space Demands	Body Structures
Social	Social Demands	*(For definitions, refer to Appendix F)*
Personal	Sequencing and Timing	
Spiritual	Required Actions	
Temporal	Required Body Functions	
Virtual	Required Body Structures	
(For definitions, refer to Appendix D)	*(For definitions, refer to Appendix E)*	

*Also referred to as basic activities of daily living (BADL) or personal activities of daily living (PADL).

Figure 3.1. Domain and dimensions of occupational therapy. This figure outlines the domain of occupational therapy and all of its dimensions. No dimension is more important than another.
From *Occupational Therapy Practice Framework: Domain and Process,* by the American Occupational Therapy Association, 2002, *American Journal of Occupational Therapy, 56,* 609–639. Copyright 2002 by the American Occupational Therapy Association. Adapted with permission.

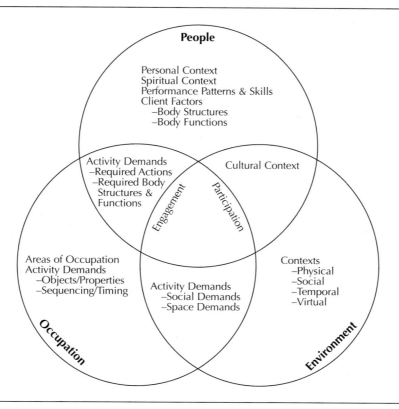

Figure 3.2. Application of the person–environment–occupation (PEO) model of occupational performance using the *Occupational Therapy Practice Framework.* This figure organizes the domain and dimensions of occupational therapy (AOTA, 2002) conceptually according to the PEO model of occupational performance (Law et al., 1996).

opportunities, employment seeking and job acquisition, work performance, and retirement planning and adjustment.

The play area of occupation refers to spontaneous or organized activities that are purely for enjoyment, entertainment, amusement, or diversion (CAOT, 1997; Parham & Fazio, 1997) and includes the exploration and social participation in these components of play. The leisure area of occupation includes "non-obligatory activity that is intrinsically motivated and engaged in during discretionary time, that is, time not committed to obligatory occupations such as work, self-care, or sleep" (Parham & Fazio, 1997, p. 250). Leisure is generally associated with freedom from work. The social participation area of occupation includes the patterns of behaviors that are characteristic and expected of an individual or an interactive collection of individuals sharing or taking part in

a social group or system. This area includes activities that result in successful interaction within communities and with society as well as with family, peers, and friends (Mosey, 1996).

Performance Skills

Addressing performance in the areas of occupation requires knowledge of the skills needed and patterns used to accomplish task components. Performance skills are actions or features of what one does (e.g., walk, choose, reach, handle), not underlying abilities, capabilities, or body functions (e.g., joint mobility, visual acuity): "Skills are observable elements of action that have implicit functional purposes" (Fisher & Kielhofner, 1995, p. 113).

There are three types of performance skills: motor, process, and communication and interaction. *Motor skills* enable people to move and interact with objects and environments and include posture, mobility, coordination, strength, and effort. *Process skills* enable people to manage and modify actions while they complete a task and include such things as energy, knowledge, temporal organization, organization of space and objects, and adaptation (Fisher & Kielhofner, 1995). *Communication and interaction skills* enable people to convey their intentions and needs as well as to orchestrate and harmonize their social behavior to interact with others. Such skills include physicality (e.g., physical contact, gestures, gazes), information exchange (e.g., asking, expressing, sharing), and relationships (e.g., collaboration, conformity) (Forsyth & Kielhofner, 1999; Forsyth, Salamy, Simon, & Kielhofner, 1997).

Performance Patterns

Performance patterns refer to the habits, routines, and roles people adopt as they engage in occupations; patterns change over time and are influenced by contexts. *Habits* are specific, automatic behaviors that are integrated into complex patterns of conduct that support or interfere with a person's ability to function on a day-to-day basis (Neistadt & Crepeau, 1998). Habits can be useful, impoverished, or dominating (Dunn, 2000). *Routines* are established sequences of occupations or activities that provide a structure for daily life, and *roles* represent "a set of behaviors that have some socially agreed upon function and for which there is an accepted code of norms" (Christiansen & Baum, 1997, p. 603). Roles organize behavior, communicate expectations, and evolve across the life span; they represent unique configurations of tasks, and some tasks fall into more than one role.

Contexts

When occupational therapy practitioners attempt to understand performance skills and patterns, they consider the contexts that influence engagement in areas of occupations. Some contexts are external to the client (e.g., physical, social, or virtual), and others are internal (e.g., personal and

spiritual). Some contexts (e.g., culture) have external features that are influenced by society and that shape internal features through indoctrination and internalization. Contexts have time dimensions, such as time of day or age (AOTA, 2002).

Activity Demands

To better understand a client's engagement in areas of occupation, practitioners also apply their analysis skills to determine the demands that a task will place on a performer and the influence of those demands on engagement and participation. Any activity involves required actions, which are dependent on performance patterns and performance skills. Furthermore, these actions place demands on body functions and structures (AOTA, 2002). Activity demands are also a function of the objects used and their properties, sequencing and timing processes, and social and space demands. Social demands external to clients place performance expectations on them, and space demands are an important environmental parameter of engagement and participation.

Client Factors

Client factors, which include body functions and structures, are attributes or foundation abilities that affect strengths and limitations in performance and ultimately engagement in occupations and participation in contexts. Body functions are the cognitive, sensory, physical, psychosocial, and affective attributes that promote or restrict engagement in occupations. Body functions involve "physiological function of body systems (including psychological functions)" (WHO, 2001, p. 10), such as mental functions (e.g., attention, memory, emotion), sensory functions (e.g., seeing, hearing, vestibular), movement-related functions (e.g., muscles, movement), and cardiovascular systems, among others. Body structures are "anatomical parts of the body such as organs, limbs, and their components" (WHO, 2001, p. 10) and include the nervous system and sensory and motor organs.

Client factors influence clients' ability to engage in occupations, and conversely engagement in occupations can also influence client factors (AOTA, 2002). For example, arthritis might limit participation in walking, but walking can help a client maintain joint mobility.

Engagement in Occupations and Participation in Contexts

The profession's primary philosophical beliefs—that engagement in occupations and participation in contexts promote health and well-being and that engagement and participation influence and are influenced by characteristics of persons, environments, and occupations—align with concepts proposed by WHO (2001). According to the ICF, health domains include human function and participation: "A person's functioning ... is conceived as a dynamic interaction between health conditions (i.e., diseases, disorders, injuries, traumas, etc.) and contextual factors" (WHO, 2001, p. 8). Participation "is an individual's involvement in life situations in relation to their health condition, body function and structures, activities, and contextual factors" (p. 14). As Law (2002a) observed, "Participation in the everyday occupations of life is a vital part of the human development and lived experience. Through participation, we acquire skills and competencies, connect with others and our communities, and find purpose and meaning in life" (p. 640). Therefore, the paradigms of the profession and WHO are connected philosophically and in practice and are used to navigate the task analysis process of evaluating persons, environments, and occupations and identifying interventions to maximize fit among them.

The Challenge

1. Define the domain of concern of occupational therapy.
2. Prepare a short list of the occupations, tasks, and activities that you find most meaningful. Occupations are self-directed, functional tasks, and activities in which a person engages over his or her life span. Tasks are a subset of occupations, and activities are the basic unit of a task (Law et al., 1996). How does engagement in the occupations, tasks, and activities you have listed lead to your personal sense of health and well-being? How does engagement in occupations enable you to participate in life situations?
3. What tasks and activities are required for engagement in the education occupation? What performance skills and patterns are required to meet the demands of these activities?
4. Examine the task (and corresponding activities) of reading a textbook. Describe the activity demands required for engagement (i.e., required actions, body structures, and body functions). What performance skills and patterns does a person need to meet these demands? How does context influence engagement in this task?
5. Identify and define the different performance patterns and skills, contexts, activity demands, and client factors that influence engagement in occupations and participation in contexts. ■

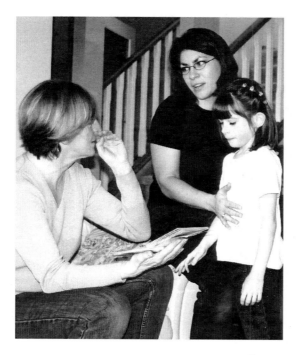

CHAPTER 4

Process of Occupational Therapy

Client-centered practice refers to collaborative approaches aimed at enabling occupation with clients who may be individuals, groups, agencies, governments, corporations, or others.

—Law, Polatajko, Baptiste, & Townsend, 1997

CHAPTER OBJECTIVES
■ To describe the relations between engagement in occupation and participation in contexts and the "fit" among people, environments, and occupations.
■ To describe the collaborative service delivery process of occupational therapy.

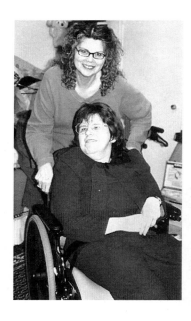

Process of Occupational Therapy

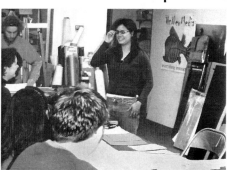

Occupational therapy practitioners see health as being shaped and influenced by the fit among the dimensions of interest to the profession, namely persons, environments, and occupations (American Occupational Therapy Association [AOTA], 1994a; Canadian Association of Occupational Therapists [CAOT], 1997; Law et al., 1996; Law, Polatajko, Baptiste, & Townsend, 1997). The person–environment–occupation (PEO) model of occupational performance clarifies this conceptualization of fit by focusing attention and analysis on the interaction and overlap among these three dimensions (Law et al., 1996). Figure 2.3 illustrates this model as containing separate but interconnected spheres that represent persons, environments, and occupations. The area where all three of the spheres overlap represents occupational performance. Engagement in occupations and participation in contexts is maximized when there is a close fit among persons, environments, and occupations. The relations among the spheres in the PEO model vary across time and are reflected in the changing performance patterns (i.e., habits, roles, routines) of persons.

An occupational performance approach to service delivery requires the use of task analysis to evaluate and maximize the dynamic, interdependent, and transactional interaction of persons, environments, and occupations. This chapter describes the process of occupational therapy proposed by AOTA (2002) and identifies parallels between this process and the PEO model of practice. The *Occupational Therapy Practice Framework: Domain and Process* (AOTA, 2002) conceptually organizes the service delivery process as illustrated in Figure 4.1, and this process has been incorporated into the occupational therapy services model in Figure 1.1. All elements of service delivery are centered on a collaborative process between practitioner and client and occur in contexts (AOTA, 2002, p. 614).

Collaborative Service Delivery Process

Evaluation

Occupational therapists start the service delivery process by developing an occupational profile and conducting an analysis of occupational performance (see Figure 1.1 and Figure 4.1). The occupational profile includes "information that describes the client's occupational history and experiences, patterns of daily living, interests, values and needs" (AOTA, 2002, p. 616). The occupational

---

▩ Evaluation

Occupational profile—The initial step in the evaluation process that provides an understanding of the client's occupational history and experiences, patterns of daily living, interests, values, and needs. The client's problems and concerns about performing occupations and daily life activities are identified, and the client's priorities are determined.

Analysis of occupational performance—The step in the evaluation process during which the client's assets, problems, or potential problems are more specifically identified. Actual performance is often observed in context to identify what supports performance and what hinders performance. Performance skills, performance patterns, context or contexts, activity demands, and client factors are all considered, but only selected aspects may be specifically assessed. Targeted outcomes are identified.

▩ Intervention

Intervention plan—A plan that will guide actions taken and that is developed in collaboration with the client. It is based on selected theories, frames of reference, and evidence. Outcomes to be targeted are confirmed.

Intervention implementation—Ongoing actions taken to influence and support improved client performance. Interventions are directed at identified outcomes. Client's response is monitored and documented.

Intervention review—A review of the implementation plan and process as well as its progress toward targeted outcomes.

▩ Outcomes (Engagement in Occupation to Support Participation)

Outcomes—Determination of success in reaching desired targeted outcomes. Outcome assessment information is used to plan future actions with the client and to evaluate the service program (i.e., program evaluation).

Figure 4.1. Framework for a collaborative service delivery process. This framework emphasizes the interactive nature of both the client–practitioner relationship and the service delivery process.
From *Occupational Therapy Practice Framework: Domain and Process,* by the American Occupational Therapy Association, 2002, *American Journal of Occupational Therapy, 56,* 609–639. Copyright 2002 by the American Occupational Therapy Association. Reprinted with permission.

profile indicates the duration and intensity of the evaluation process, and client priorities guide the focus of the evaluation and the analysis of occupational performance in particular. In addition, the occupational profile enables the occupational therapist to develop "a working hypothesis regarding possible reasons for identified problems and concerns, and identifies the client's strengths and weaknesses" (AOTA, 2002, p. 617). The practitioner uses this information to better understand the client and his or her desired levels of participation and to identify areas in which intervention is needed to enhance engagement in occupations.

During the evaluation process, occupational therapists also conduct an analysis of occupational performance to more clearly specify the client's assets, problems, and potential problems. The practitioner considers performance skills, performance patterns, context or contexts, activity demands, and client factors, but he or she may specifically assess only selected aspects deemed relevant because they contribute to or limit occupational perform-

ance (AOTA, 2002). The therapist does not formulate a "diagnosis"; he or she simply describes and analyzes the client's circumstances and contexts in relation to engagement and participation.

Occupational performance analysis focuses on characteristics of persons and their engagement in occupations and participation in contexts. The client's assets, problems, or potential problems are identified, levels of participation and engagement may be observed, and dimensions of performance evaluated. Targeted outcomes are then identified (AOTA, 2002). When the client is an individual, the practitioner maps the client's participation in areas of occupation and the relevance and meaningfulness of different tasks and activities relative to performance. When the client is a group, the practitioner seeks to identify variations in levels of participation and coherence and synergies among its members. When the client is a population, occupational performance analysis involves profiling participation rates (e.g., proportion of persons with disabilities who are

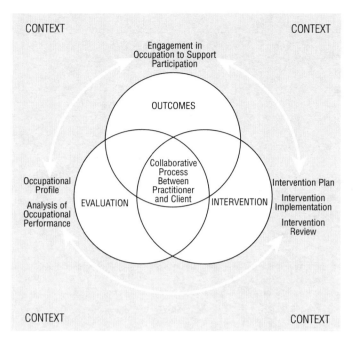

Figure 4.2. Framework Collaborative Process Model. Illustration of the framework emphasizing client–practitioner interactive relationship and interactive nature of the service delivery process.

From *Occupational Therapy Practice Framework: Domain and Process,* by the American Occupational Therapy Association, 2002, *American Journal of Occupational Therapy, 56,* 609–639. Copyright 2002 by the American Occupational Therapy Association. Reprinted with permission.

employed) using data about the population that are available or that the practitioner gathers.

The analysis process focuses on the person and occupation dimensions (i.e., activity demands) that influence engagement and participation (see Figure 4.2). When the client is an individual, the dimensions of interest include the following:

• performance skills,
• performance patterns,
• personal and spiritual contexts,
• client factors, and
• activity demands.

When services are directed toward populations of people, the characteristics of interest include

• health indicators;
• the lifestyles of the community or cohort of people;

• sociocultural values;
• prevalence, incidence, and temporal trends in impairments, conditions, and risk behaviors; and
• commitment to and preparedness for change.

In addition, the analysis of occupational performance focuses on environmental factors that contribute to, support, or hinder participation, such as the cultural, physical, social, temporal, and virtual contexts and the social and space aspects of activity demands.

Through the process of assessing the interactions among these dimensions, the occupational therapist identifies target outcomes and determines priorities in collaboration with clients or their proxies. The evaluation process thus sets the stage for intervention.

Intervention

The collaborative relationship between occupational therapy practitioners and clients is the foundation for intervention planning, implementation, and review. The intervention process begins with a plan to maximize the fit between clients and their environments and occupations (see Figure 1.1). Evaluation has considered client factors, activity demands, and contextual determinants of engagement in occupation, so the occupational therapy practitioner can target intervention at any one or more of these dimensions to facilitate participation. The intervention plan, which guides the actions taken, is developed in collaboration with the client. This process is referred to as "client-centered" as the client directs the service.

Intervention implementation is the process of undertaking actions to influence, support, build, and strengthen client capacity to engage in occupations and participate in contexts. The occupational therapist selects services guided by theories, frames of reference, clinical reasoning, and research evidence regarding the effectiveness of specific services for certain clientele. There are five occupational therapy approaches based on theory and evidence: (a) create or promote, (b) establish or restore, (c) maintain, (d) modify or adapt, and (e) prevent; these approaches are defined in Appendix G (refer also to Figure 1.1).

The health promotion approach to intervention is designed to create enriched contextual and activity experiences to enhance engagement and participation of all people in the natural contexts of life. The restorative approach seeks to establish skills or abilities in clients that have not yet been developed. The maintenance approach is designed to provide supports that enable clients to preserve levels of engagement and participation. The adaptation approach is directed toward modifying contexts or activity demands to support engagement and participation in natural contexts. Finally, the prevention approach is designed to minimize risk of disability and to prevent barriers to engagement and participation.

The *Occupational Therapy Practice Framework* describes four modes of intervention: (a) therapeutic use of self, (b) therapeutic use of occupations and activities, (c) consultation, and (d) education, defined in Appendix H. *Therapeutic use of self* refers to a practitioner's planned use of his or her personality, communication skills, interaction style, insights, perceptions, and judgments to facilitate the therapy process. Hagedorn (1997) noted that "the basic skills of listening, observing non-verbal cues and adapting responses are required by all health care practitioners" (p. 21). *Therapeutic use of occupations and activities* includes occupation-based activity, purposeful activity, and preparatory methods. *Occupation-based activity* is used to enable clients to engage in actual occupations in their own contexts to address goals of intervention. By comparison, *purposeful activity* facilitates clients' engagement in goal-directed behaviors or activities within a therapeutically designed context. *Preparatory methods,* such as the use of exercise or assistive devices, prepare clients for engagement in purposeful activities or occupation-based activities.

The *consultation process* involves practitioners applying their knowledge and expertise to collaboration with the client. In the *education process,* the practitioner imparts knowledge and information through interventions such as instruction and teaching with individuals and groups and health education initiatives targeted toward communities and populations. Occupational therapy practitioners who engage in academic teaching and scholarly writing teach others strategies to improve the health of their clients.

The occupational therapist continuously reviews the effectiveness of intervention in bringing about progress toward established goals. The therapist monitors and documents progress, and the implementation plan is appraised through this process of intervention review.

Outcomes

Early in the intervention process, practitioners and clients select the areas of occupation and levels of engagement in these areas that will become the expected outcomes of services. Achieving successful outcomes of occupational therapy services depends on success in achieving predefined client goals and objectives. Although engagement in occupation to support participation in context (i.e., occupational performance) is the primary targeted outcome, other outcomes of service delivery include client satisfaction, role competence, adaptation, healthy lifestyles, quality of life, and health and wellness (see Figure 1.1). These occupational therapy outcomes are defined in Appendix I.

The instrument or instruments used to measure and track progress are selected on the basis of psychometric properties such as validity, reliability, and sensitivity to change. Outcome assessment information can be used to evaluate the effectiveness of both an intervention strategy and a model of service delivery. While this text focuses on the identification of priority client outcomes, readers who seek to better understand the measurement of occupational therapy outcomes are encouraged to review Forer (1996) and Watson (2000).

The Challenge

1. One of the first stages in developing an occupational profile is to develop an understanding of the client's occupational history, patterns of daily living, interests, values, and needs. Develop open-ended questions that could be used to guide an interview process designed to collect this type of information from clients.

2. Practice the interview process with a partner.

   a. Consider the importance of communicating well in the initial stages of the client–practitioner relationship. Davis (1989) noted that "first impressions very often count, and the importance of obtaining a patient's trust from the outset of [the] interaction together is invaluable to the healing process" (p. 103).

   b. Get feedback from your partner on how you phrased and timed questions throughout the interview process. Practice rephrasing questions to improve your approach. Did you listen carefully and project a good level of attention and involvement? Did you avoid jargon and slang?

3. After the interview, organize the key points into a concise summary of the occupational performance of the person interviewed.

   a. Have your partner confirm if the profile is congruent with the information he or she provided in the interview.

   b. Identify where your value systems may have led you to interpret information incorrectly.

4. Describe the similarities and differences in the occupational therapy process when services are directed toward individuals and toward populations. ■

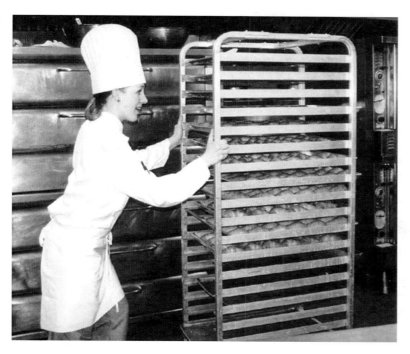

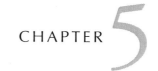

CHAPTER 5

Serving Individuals and Populations

An occupational performance approach to evaluation and intervention focuses on the dynamic, interdependent, and transactional relations among people in communities, their typical occupations and actions, and the community and societal contexts in which they live. This is true whether services are directed at individuals, communities, or populations.

CHAPTER OBJECTIVE
■ Describe the occupational therapy service delivery process for individuals and for populations.

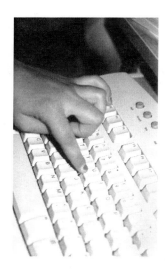

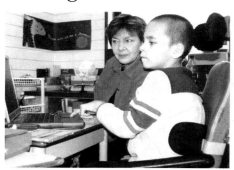

Serving Individuals and Populations

Changes in the nature and distribution of health and risk of ill health, coupled with an enhanced understanding of the determinants of health and illness, have altered the nature of demand for the services health practitioners provide. Occupational therapy practitioners now offer services not only to individual clients who seek to alter their levels of engagement and participation but also to populations of persons who seek to alter their levels of health and well-being. In all instances, occupational therapy practitioners target evaluation and intervention to optimizing the interactions among persons, environments, and occupations. Because people are members of groups, organizations, communities, and populations, the art and science of occupational therapy are applicable to all of these social entities. This chapter describes the similarities and differences in the service delivery process to individuals and to populations and illustrates the use of task analysis as a clinical reasoning tool for individuals and populations.

Review of the Service Delivery Process

Occupational therapy practitioners start the service delivery process by developing an occupational profile and conducting an analysis of occupational performance. Task analysis is used as part of occupational performance analysis to assess the contribution of performance skills, performance patterns, contexts, activity demands, and client factors to engagement and participation (American Occupational Therapy Association [AOTA], 2002). Additionally, task analysis helps occupational therapy practitioners determine which occupations, tasks, and activities a particular client must perform to assume a lifestyle or level of participation that he or she values. Task analysis enables practitioners to determine how an impairment or disability influences engagement and participation and to make predictions about potential future gains in functional levels (Mattingly & Flemming, 1994). This determination assists the practitioner in structuring and streamlining the evaluation process and may help clients make more informed decisions regarding the need for intervention.

Occupational therapists and clients collaborate during the evaluation process to identify intervention goals and priorities. Clients describe or demonstrate the meaningful occupations that they have difficulty with but would like to perform. The therapist uses task analysis, clinical observations, and formal and standardized assessments to evaluate the dimensions of occupational performance; conceptual frameworks and theoretical frames of reference give the process direction and coherence (Mosey, 1981).

Intervention planning occurs after the initial evaluation and subsequent identification of the client's long-term goals and short-term objectives. Long-term goals relate to activity limitations in areas of occupation that clients want addressed. Short-term objectives relate to the performance skills and patterns and client factors that must be altered, modified, or augmented and environmental parameters that must be addressed for the client to achieve the long-term goals. Task analysis may be used to divide long-term goals into smaller, measurable units of activity. In essence, these goals define the dimensions in which outcomes are sought. It is progress toward these goals that clients will monitor and therapists will measure. By measuring progress toward targeted outcomes, therapists are assessing the intervention plan and implementation to ensure that it is effective.

Occupational therapy practitioners direct intervention services at maximizing the fit between the person (i.e., client) and his or her environments (i.e., contexts) and occupations, and task analysis is used by practitioners to determine whether to target intervention to the person (e.g., remedial, maintenance, compensation), occupation (e.g., alteration of activity demands), or context (e.g., health promotion, disability prevention). Intervention directed at enabling people to develop the foundational abilities to support performance and participation includes (a) restoring, remediating, or maintaining performance skills and client factors; (b) teaching new methods or compensation strategies through practice opportunities; and (c) promoting new performance patterns, lifestyles, or ways of living through educational approaches. Intervention directed at the occupation includes (a) enabling clients to practice occupation-based activities to promote participation, mastery, and self-esteem; (b) helping clients engage in purposeful activities to develop or improve performance skills and client factors; and (c) altering activity demands to promote success. When intervention must address

both personal and environmental contexts, it may include modifying or altering environments and promoting healthy attitudes that foster participation, prevent injury, and minimize the disabling effects of impairments.

Purposeful activities are an intervention that translates theories, models, approaches, and strategies into concrete activities that promote skills and adaptation (Hagedorn, 1997; Trombly, 1995b). On the basis of activity analysis, practitioners can design intrinsically rewarding, meaningful, and therapeutic activities that balance situational challenges with personal skills (Csikszentmihalyi, 1990). Purposeful activities are therapeutic when they (a) are relevant, meaningful, and goal directed; (b) elicit coordination among sensorimotor, cognitive, psychological, and psychosocial systems; and (c) promote mastery and feelings of self-competence (AOTA, 1993; Fidler & Fidler, 1978; Trombly, 1995a). Activity analysis can also help practitioners determine alternative ways for clients to participate in their contexts that may involve modifying activity demands.

Practitioners who are skilled at activity and task analysis are able to select the most appropriate activity from among those of interest to a particular client (Trombly, 1995b) or to modify an activity that a client has selected to optimize its therapeutic value. Activity has been used as a treatment modality since the early years of occupational therapy practice, and the use of therapeutic activity to improve performance skills and patterns is "based on the assumption that the activity holds within itself a healing property that will change organic or behavioral impairments" (Trombly, 1995a, p. 964). In this context, engagement in purposeful activities has the potential to restore or remediate client factors as well as performance skills and patterns.

Mattingly and Flemming (1994) recommended that practitioners think about the whole condition, including the person, the activity limitation, the meanings the activity limitation has for the person, the person's roles and responsibilities, and the impact of performance limitations on significant others. This process of conditional reasoning enables occupational therapy practitioners to envision a client's potential. The realization of that potential, however, is conditional on its compatibility with the client's own construction of a vision for the future. Therefore, practitioners must enlist clients' participation in this process by suggesting meaningful choices during treatment and by structuring therapeutic activities to address multiple, simultaneous, and individualized goals. Task analysis is used throughout the process to determine appropriate intervention strategies to address the aims of service provision based on the client's occupational goals. Clients are typically discharged when they achieve their maximum potential as measured by goal attainment.

When services are directed toward groups of individuals, practitioners evaluate each group member and design cohesive intervention plans to address the goals and objectives of all the individuals within the group. Interventions may be targeted toward improving participation and health among all individuals within a group and reducing risk of activity limitations and participation restrictions (AOTA, 2002). Group-based services focus on the practitioner's use of self to create an environment that will support change among members. Purposeful activities completed within the group promote performance skills and develop or restore client factors required for enhanced engagement in occupations. Remedial interventions used in groups, therefore, include the practitioners' therapeutic use of self, purposeful activities, and the facilitation of group process and interactions (Donohue & Greer, 2000). Task analysis during evaluation enables practitioners to monitor the dynamic interactions among group members and the purposeful activities in which they are engaged to promote group cohesion and attainment of individual outcomes. Although interventions are directed at the group level, it is the individuals within the group who are being served. If the group is not cohesive around goals and objectives that are driven by individual clients, the group may not facilitate individual change toward desired outcomes.

Service Delivery to Populations

Although the most common form of service delivery involves services directed toward individual clients, more and more health practitioners serve populations. Populations can be defined on the basis of geography (e.g., neighborhoods, communities) or shared characteristics (e.g., students, older adults, workers, members of an organization). Population-based services focus on the "needs of a group of individuals as a whole rather than on the specific needs of an individual" (Moyers, 1999, p. 263).

In 2000 the U.S. Department of Health and Human Services (DHHS) outlined a comprehensive, nationwide agenda to improve the health of the U.S. population that addressed the needs of individuals as a collective. The *Healthy People 2010* agenda includes health goals, objectives, and indicators that are "grounded in science, built through public consensus, and designed to measure progress" (DHHS, 2000, p. 1). The underlying premise of *Healthy People 2010,* which is based on an in-depth review of research, is that the health of individuals is inseparable from the health of the larger community and that it is the health of every community that determines the overall health of the nation. Likewise, the health of communities is profoundly influenced by the collective behaviors, actions, attitudes, and beliefs of the persons who live in them. Like the national plan to improve the health of the nation, occupational therapy intervention plans are designed to improve the health of individuals or populations and must also be grounded in science, built in collaboration with clients, and designed to address targeted outcomes. Interestingly, the dimensions of concern identified in *Healthy People 2010* as the determinants of the population's health are strikingly similar to the dimensions of concern to occupational therapy practitioners. (These parallels are described more thoroughly in chapter 15.) And, whereas health status is seen by the DHHS (2000) as a function of the interaction of people and environments, participation in occupations is seen by AOTA (2002) as a function of people and contexts.

When providing services to populations, practitioners first profile the needs, assets, and priorities of the people (i.e., occupational profile). They do this by establishing collaborative relationships with individuals who serve as proxies for the collective and who are empowered to direct the course of intervention. Needs are defined on the basis of discrepancies between current and desired levels of engagement in occupations, and disparities in attainment of desired levels of participation among groups within the population must be considered when identifying needs. *Assets* are the inherent attributes and available resources of populations that might be used in attaining target outcomes. An analysis of the occupational performance of populations requires an understanding of the people (e.g., health status indicators; prevalence, incidence, and temporal trends in impairments; health conditions and risk behaviors; performance patterns or lifestyles), occupations (e.g., activity demands), and environments (e.g., social and cultural contexts).

The occupational profile and occupational performance analysis form the basis for the development of intervention goals, objectives, priorities, and initiatives, which become the vision, mission, and guiding principles embedded in service delivery mechanisms and community-based development processes. The evaluation and intervention processes are always client directed in that services focus on the priorities identified by clients or their proxies.

When services are directed toward improving the health of populations, intervention is targeted toward people and environmental contexts to promote engagement in occupations and support participation in contexts. Intervention may be designed to create enabling contexts (i.e., health promotion) or to reduce activity limitations among persons with impairments (i.e., disease and disability prevention). This process requires an educational and consultative approach to services: "Community partnerships, particularly when they reach out to non-traditional partners, can be among the most effective tools for improving health in communities" (DHHS, 2000, p. 4).

Whereas services directed toward individuals often reflect a medical or behavioral model of care, health services directed at communities and populations tend to be behavioral and socioenvironmental in nature. The medical model focuses on health as the absence of disease. The focus of intervention is to target high-risk or high-need individuals and manage disease and impairment through physiological means (e.g., immunization programs, pharmaceutical management). Behavioral models focus on individual responsibility for correcting unhealthy behaviors through positive lifestyle change. The intent is to reduce behavioral risk factors (e.g., smoking, poor nutrition, insufficient physical activity) in individuals or among individuals in a population.

Behavioral models of intervention are intended to influence people by altering their physical, social, and cultural contexts. These interventions focus on health education (e.g., messages that smoking is bad for one's health), social marketing (e.g., messages that smoking among mothers endangers unborn children or that secondhand smoking endangers the health of others), and public policy (e.g., smoking is illegal for underage individuals or not allowed in public locations). Health behaviors, however, are notoriously hard to change. Decisions to smoke, drink, engage in unsafe sex, and so forth are not simply matters of rational choice but are embedded in complex social contexts. Public health efforts have reduced the prevalence of smoking, drunk driving, and other unhealthy behaviors, but monumental change in the behavior of populations requires more than increased knowledge, persuasion, or health education; people engage in substance abuse even when they are aware of the health consequences. Research also suggests that behavioral models have differential impacts on different segments of the population and that intervention has not satisfactorily achieved targeted outcomes in some segments. For example, smoking continues to be more prevalent among women than men, among teenagers than adults, and among low-socioeconomic populations than higher-socioeconomic groups.

When intervention is targeted toward environmental contexts, *socioenvironmental* or *ecological models* are used to focus services on broad determinants of the health of the population, including physical, social, cultural, institutional, political, and virtual environments (AOTA, 2002; World Health Organization [WHO], 2001). The intent is to reduce impediments to health and provide opportunities for health by influencing policies and interventions, access to health care, and community-directed change (DHHS, 2000; Labonte, 1993; McBeth & Schweer, 2000). Occupational therapy practitioners can and do influence public policy and design and offer prevention and health promotion services to influence the population's level of participation in meaningful occupations. For example, occupational therapy practitioners have been involved in drafting and revising federal legislation governing the educational rights of persons with disabilities. They have been involved in designing and evaluating prevention programs to enhance capacity for successful aging by using consultative and educational intervention approaches to help older people better appreciate and engage in meaningful occupations (Clarke et al., 1997, 2001; Hay et al., 2002). Insofar as city councils or regional governing bodies are designing or altering local and national policies and programs that influence resources for health and participation in occupations, there is a role for occupational therapy practitioners. The fundamental conditions and resources for health defined by the WHO (2001), which include peace, shelter, education, food, income, a stable ecosystem, sustainable resources, social justice, and equity, are all amenable to socioenvironmental intervention by occupational therapy practitioners.

There is not necessarily a direct relation between disability and health; many persons with disabilities rate their health as excellent. Therefore, health practitioners are shifting their focus from evaluation and intervention for clients with disabilities to the provision of services to persons who have activity limitations and participation restrictions that result in undesirable states of health. Furthermore, the prevalence of disability is increasing and can be expected to accelerate in the coming decades as the population ages and medical technology advances. Most recent estimates are that one-fifth of Americans, or 50 million people, have a disability (McNeil, 2001). Health interventions, therefore, are increasingly being targeted to communities and are focusing on health promotion and disability prevention. For example, health interventions are being designed to enable communities to build and strengthen multisectoral partnerships to promote healthy lifestyles and improve the health and social conditions in the places people live, work, and play. The healthy communities concept, which has its origins in seminal documents published in Canada and the United States, is a strategy WHO (1980) has recommended to strengthen health promotion activities in regions. This strategy integrates public health, health education, and community development.

Occupational therapy practitioners can and should integrate medical, behavioral, and socioenvironmental models into their practice. All of these models have had, and continue to have, a role in enabling health, engagement in occupations, and participation in contexts. Medical models are appropriate to use when the focus is on altering or minimizing impairments to reduce risk of disability. Behavioral models are appropriate to use when the focus is on changing the lifestyles of individuals or populations. Socioenvironmental models are appropriate to address the broader, contextual determinants of health. Whether services are directed toward individuals, groups, communities, or populations, occupational therapy evaluation and intervention always focus on understanding and promoting the alignment or fit among persons, environments, and occupations. Collaborative relationships with clients and their proxies, client-directed services, and partnerships with stakeholders who are interested in similar target outcomes remain the constant foundation of the occupational therapy process.

Practice with individuals, groups, communities, and populations has provided evidence for the robust ability of the profession's theories, knowledge base, practice models, and intervention approaches to enable clients to engage in occupations and participate in contexts. By reflecting on the interventions they have used in their practice with individual clients, practitioners can learn more about what interventions can enable populations to engage in occupations and participate in contexts. The case study of Scott illustrates how occupational therapy practitioners can use task analysis in providing services to individuals, groups, and populations. The case study also demonstrates the domain and process of occupational therapy practice with different types of clientele.

The Challenge

1. Describe the similarities and differences of the occupational therapy service delivery process when services are directed toward individuals and toward populations.
2. Review the Client Profile and Task Analysis Form in Appendix J to become familiar with the dimensions of evaluation in the development of an occupational profile. ■

CASE STUDY: SCOTT
Work With Individuals

Scott was an occupational therapy practitioner working at ABC Rehabilitation Center, a facility providing inpatient, outpatient, and community-based services. He had extensive experience in work with clients who have had traumatic injuries, and one of his clients was Ann.[1] Ann was a single mother who recently had had her right arm amputated just below the elbow following an injury in a commercial kitchen. Her initial priorities related to returning to her roles as a mother of two young boys, homemaker, worker, and sole provider. Ann was particularly concerned about her ability to return to her job as a chef's assistant.

Ann and Scott agreed that improvements in levels of participation in basic activities of daily living

(ADL) (e.g., dressing, personal hygiene), instrumental activities of daily living (IADL) (e.g., meal preparation and cleanup), leisure (playing with sons, sewing), and social participation (family, peers, community interaction) were necessary for re-entry into the workforce. Scott completed an evaluation, and he and Ann worked together to establish client goals and objectives.

Ann was discouraged by the amount of time and effort required for ADL and her lack of independence in this area. Scott observed Ann dressing and applying makeup and determined that she had not developed proficiency with the prosthesis (a motor performance skill). Furthermore, all of her blouses had buttons, her cosmetic bag had a small zipper, and her makeup containers were very small and delicate (activity demands); all required a higher level of manipulative skill than Ann was capable of performing.

Using task analysis, Scott determined that activity demands (e.g.,

small zippers and containers), contextual dimensions (e.g., recent injury, lack of spouse, not wanting children to assist with personal care), and performance skill dimensions (e.g., dexterity) were causing participation restrictions and frustrating limitations. Scott used his analytic skills to determine which areas of dressing would be addressed first to ensure that Ann attained success rapidly. On the basis of ongoing task analysis and consultation with Ann, Scott modified and expanded the initial objectives in the area of dressing over time to ensure success in progressively more difficult activities. Once they agreed on goals, Scott elected to use a remedial approach to developing performance skills and a compensatory approach to modifying activity demands. He expected to utilize therapeutic use of self, therapeutic use of occupations and activities, consultation, and education.

Scott explored Ann's interest in a number of IADL and leisure activities,

---

[1]The client cases in this book depict hypothetical events and are intended to serve as a basis for learning. Any similarities to real persons or events are purely coincidental.

including baking, sewing, typing, and writing letters (handwriting was also a work-related activity). Ann decided to try baking cookies and sewing. During initial baking sessions, Scott encouraged Ann to practice manipulating all of the ingredients and utensils (i.e., preparatory method). Scott determined, using his task analysis skills, that Ann was easily frustrated by her inability to adjust to the lack of upper-limb sensory information (i.e., client factors) that she relied on before the amputation. This caused her to drop objects she held in her right prosthesis when she directed her vision and attention elsewhere (i.e., performance skill). Ann was frustrated by her inability to work with both hands to bake and sew. She needed to learn safe practices associated with heat when baking and the rapidly moving sewing machine needle to prevent secondary injury. Scott realized he needed to enrich his intervention plan to include a prevention approach.

Scott used task analysis to determine that Ann's ability to control the bowl when stirring cooking ingredients was insufficient and made a clinical judgment that this task would remain difficult until she was more proficient with the prosthesis. He suggested modifying the work surface through the use of nonslip matting to keep the bowl from sliding while Ann mixed ingredients and formed cookies (i.e., alter activity demands). As Ann's coordination and manipulative performance skills improved (through remedial use of therapeutic occupations and activi-

ties), she progressed to practicing opening and closing containers. When she was still unable to open the package of chocolate chips, Scott showed her how to use modified scissors (alteration of activity demands, education as an intervention). Likewise, Ann was pleased to find that she could use a sewing machine by slowing the speed of the machine and consciously directing the flow of the fabric using her left hand and the hook of her right prosthesis (adaptation).

Ann relearned how to sew using her prosthesis by making a cosmetic bag with a drawstring and sewing hook-and-loop fasteners on the fronts of her shirts. Engagement in sewing improved her proficiency with the prosthesis, and completion of these projects eliminated the need for Ann to master shirt button closures or a small cosmetic bag zipper. She thus gained independence with dressing, makeup management, and sewing. Eventually, Ann began to envision herself actively participating in the important roles in her life: mother, homemaker, and worker.

Through the individualized therapy process, Ann eventually gained greater independence in ADL, IADL, and work activities. Once she was discharged, the daily patterns of her life began to be reestablished. Before discharge from inpatient rehabilitation, Ann participated in a return-to-work program. Scott helped Ann recognize how the intervention process had prepared her to return to work. During group therapy, she discussed

potential problems that may emerge at her workplace, and she was able to discuss her fear of returning to work with some of her colleagues. When she was discharged, she felt prepared to meet unexpected challenges.

Work With Groups

Scott completed evaluations of three adults who were referred for occupational therapy services following a motor vehicle accident or workplace injury. (Ann was one of these clients.) After completing an occupational profile and occupational performance analysis for each client, he realized that they would likely face similar challenges returning to work. Armed with this information and insight, he approached all three clients to determine their interest in meeting as a group to work on workplace performance skills. Scott proposed several potential therapeutic activities they could do together (e.g., planning a menu and hosting a luncheon) to simultaneously address common adaptation issues and individualized goals (e.g., performance skills). For example, Ann could direct group activities using the performance skills related to the demands of her job (e.g., preparing and carrying plates of food). Scott relied on using the intervention approach of therapeutic use of self to guide discussions around adaptation. He used task analysis and clinical reasoning to guide decisions regarding alterations of activity demands to address the different individualized goals of the clients participating in the group.

Work With Populations

Over the years Scott had worked with individual clients, populations of workers, and industry. In his practice with injured workers, employers and insurers often asked him to determine how best to get an individual worker back on the job and to provide recommendations for altering job demands and environmental conditions to prevent further injuries at the site. Scott realized that many of the recommendations he made to prevent workplace injury for an individual applied to the population of workers. These recommendations tended to be derived from his experience working with people such as Ann, who had upper limb amputations following a workplace injury. In fact, Scott's clientele represented a portion of the population of people in the United States with these types of injury.

Scott was among a group of practitioners in the country who were contacted by researchers to assist in an important project by collecting data about his clientele. The research goal was to describe the population of individuals with upper-limb amputations resulting from workplace injury, accurately estimate their occupational outcomes, and identify factors that contributed to successful recovery following injury. Before developing a return-to-work program for his clients, Scott completed a review of the literature to evaluate evidence regarding effective intervention strategies. To his disappointment, there was not a substantial body of high-quality research in this area. He hoped that by con-

tributing to this study, the evidence generated would assist him and other practitioners in identifying the most effective approaches to workplace injury prevention and rehabilitation. This evidence would enable Scott and others to target prevention occupational therapy services.

Scott was approached by a member of the Chamber of Commerce, who had learned about him and his work through Ann. Many members of the Chamber were becoming increasingly concerned about workplace injury, and they wanted to do something about it. When they approached Scott, he wondered why he had not thought of working with them before. He was very enthusiastic about the possibilities of designing health interventions with them to reduce risk of injury and promote successful adaptation among those who are injured. After attending a meeting of the Chamber, Scott hypothesized that most of the work injuries described were preventable. He decided to meet with a focus group of health care practitioners from the local emergency department and a group of general practitioners to more fully understand the issues.

Members of the Chamber, Scott, and some of his colleagues set out to determine the characteristics of the population of workers in their community and their work contexts to profile their needs and assets and establish priorities. One member of the Chamber was familiar with obtaining and using information from

the Census Bureau, and Scott volunteered to contact the regional health department to solicit their partnership in this initiative. Scott and his team searched out information on the incidence of workplace injury, the incidence of mortality due to injury, the prevalence of morbidity due to injury, characteristics of those most at risk for injury, the level of knowledge among employers regarding risk factors for injury, and other useful data. The team collected data on the most frequent causes of injury among workers, current levels of engagement of employees in these activities, and contextual factors that may influence rates of injury and morbidity following injury (e.g., job site orientation, safety and maintenance of workplace equipment, injury prevention programs).

On the basis of current and relevant information and his expertise in task analysis, Scott recommended that the Chamber engage the community and all employers in initiatives that their research findings suggested would potentially have the greatest impact on the rates of workplace injury and resulting morbidity. Knowing that the insights he has gained from the population health data would be of great interest to and arouse great concern among others, Scott worked with the Chamber to create an intersectoral and interdisciplinary coalition of individuals from the community to develop an action plan that would address the full scope of factors that contributed to the prevention of injury in the workplace.

This coalition eventually consisted of stakeholder representatives from the profit, not-for-profit, and volunteer sectors, as well as local and state government.

Scott, acting as a committee member for the coalition, worked with employers and other members of the team to partner with several organizations and industries in their community to design educational materials to inform the community about the prevalence and incidence of the problem, about the economic impact and burden of illness following workplace injury, and about behaviors that put people at risk of injury while at work. The objective of the material was to stimulate individual and community action to alter risk behaviors, maximize compliance with legislation designed to reduce risk of injury (e.g., laws that required construction workers to wear helmets), and alter physical environments that placed workers at risk, such as cluttered work spaces. The newly formed coalition merged health promotion initiatives with those designed to prevent injury in the workplace, such as enhancing the safety of the job sites associated with the highest rates of injury; increasing the availability of first aid, ambulance, and emergency services; ensuring that medical and rehabilitation services were directed toward minimizing activity limitations among workers with injury-related impairments; and promoting industry-supported fitness programs. ∎

Health of Individuals and Groups

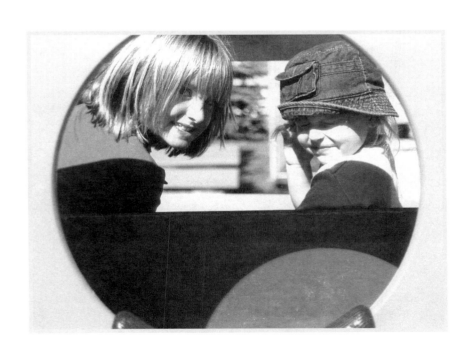

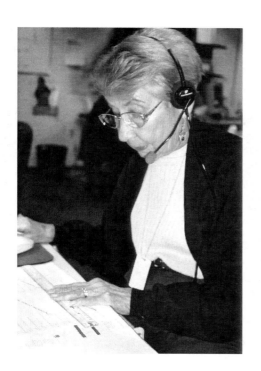

 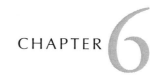
Occupations Over the Life Span

Occupational therapy practitioners' focus on helping people engage in occupations and participate in contexts extends across the life span.

CHAPTER OBJECTIVES
- To review the life span transitions that influence engagement in occupations and participation in contexts.
- To show how the dynamic interaction among persons, environments, and occupations is consistent across the life span.

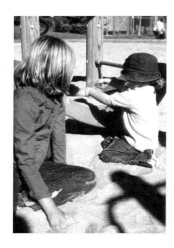

Occupations Over the Life Span

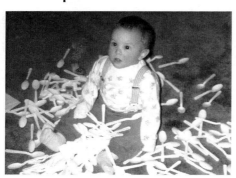

Life span transitions influence engagement in occupations and participation in contexts. Newborns begin to develop performance skills (e.g., feeding) and patterns (e.g., routines) during the first few days following their birth, and young infants engage in increasingly complex occupations through participation in activities of daily living (ADL), social interactions, and play. These daily life occupations provide tremendous opportunities for learning during the early years; these experiences lay the foundation for further refinement of performance skills and patterns during preschool years and for acquisition of knowledge and application of skills during the school years. Engagement in occupations during childhood leads to the development of identity, social skills, emotional well-being, and prevocational pursuits in adolescence, and later to the vocational pursuits and expanded diversity of social interactions in adulthood. Because the maintenance of health and well-being during older adulthood seems to be predicated on developmental and occupational history, among other things, occupational therapy practitioners require an understanding of life span trajectories and transitions.

Childhood Occupations

The role of occupational therapy practitioners who work with children and collaborate with parents, caregivers, and other stakeholders is to enhance children's engagement in their occupations and participation in their contexts. Practitioners seek to support the daily life activities of children, which include ADL, play, education, social participation, and leisure. Examples of developmental expectations of children in different areas of occupation are provided in Table 6.1, and this information will contribute to readers' understanding of the case studies in chapters 7–11.

Occupational therapy practitioners first evaluate individual children or the status of a population of children to identify underlying performance skills and patterns, as well as contexts, activity demands, and client factors (both internal and external to the client) that support or limit participation in areas of occupation. The purposes of the evaluation process are to profile occupational history and identify interests, values, and needs; analyze activity demands and contextual characteristics; and understand the concerns of the family, school, and community. For an individual child, primary sources of information for an occupational profile

Table 6.1. Developmental expectations for children, by area of occupation.

Area of Occupation	Task	Expected Developmental Activity
Activities of daily living	Dressing	Puts on socks, shoes, and shorts at age 2 years Ties shoe laces at 5–6 years Needs help with buttons and right or left shoe at 3 years Knows front and back of clothing at 4 years Buttons (4.5 years) and unbuttons (4 years) front-opening garments Zips up front-opening clothing at 5 years
	Education	Cuts paper with scissors at 3 years Cuts curved lines and simple shapes at 5 years Draws a recognizable face at 4–5 years Can do palmar pencil grasp at 1–2 years, static tripod grasp at 3–4 years, and dynamic tripod grasp at 4–6 years Draws circles at 3 years, squares at 4.5 years, and triangles at 5 years Matches objects and primary colors at 3 years Counts to three at 4 years
	Play or leisure	Catches large ball from 5 feet at 2.5–3 years Catches small ball at approximately 3 years Throws overhand 3 feet at 1.5–2 years Kicks a stationary ball at 3 years Rides a tricycle without pedals at 1.5–2 years Uses tricycle pedals to propel tricycle at 2.5–3 years
	Social participation	Tells names of friends and relatives at 3–4 years Is adamant about making own decisions at 2–3 years Engages in parallel play at 1.5–2 years, cooperative play at > 2 years, and interactive play at > 3 years Behaves according to peer group norm at 4–5 years

are interviews with parents, teachers, and other caregivers. The occupational therapy practitioner also observes actual performance in the child's customary environments to identify the contextual components that support or hinder engagement in occupations. Finally, standardized and informal evaluation tools can help occupational therapists confirm their hypotheses regarding performance skills and patterns and client factors that contribute to or hinder engagement and participation.

In collaboration with parents, day care, preschool, school staff members, and other stakeholders, practitioners then develop intervention plans to address target outcomes for their pediatric clients. Remediation or restoration and compensation or adaptation are effective approaches to intervention with individuals. Remediation and restoration seek to challenge clients to estab-

lish skills or abilities that they have not yet developed or to restore a skill or ability that has been impaired (Dunn, 1998). The primary therapeutic medium used in remedial or restorative approaches to intervention with children is therapeutic play activity. When a child needs to develop particular performance skills and patterns, occupational therapy practitioners identify purposeful and therapeutic activities and artfully blend these activities into the typical daily routine of the child and family. Play delights a child and has added purpose other than entertainment and exercise. Purposeful play activities are therapeutic when they (a) are relevant, meaningful, and goal directed; (b) elicit coordination among sensorimotor, cognitive, perceptual, and psychosocial systems; and (c) promote mastery and feelings of self-competence (American Occupational Therapy

Association [AOTA], 1993, 2002; Fidler & Fidler, 1978).

Occupational therapy practitioners also use compensation and adaptation approaches to intervention to revise current contexts or activity demands and give children the opportunity to learn and practice new methods that support their engagement in occupations. The case studies of Bobbie, Tina, Miguel, Sidney, and Wayne in chapters 7–11 provide opportunities for readers to practice task analysis during evaluation and intervention with pediatric clients.

Health promotion and disability prevention approaches to intervention can be used with populations as well as with individuals. Chapters 17 and 18 describe the use of these approaches in improving the health of populations of children.

Adolescent Occupations

The decade of adolescence (ages 11–18 years) is a time of rapid change. Adolescents undergo a transition from their childhood roles of dependency and reliance on parents and others to adult roles that are marked by emotional independence from parents and personal directedness. Adolescence is also a time for further development of performance skills and patterns and alteration in body structures and functions. Adolescents continue to establish their self-identity, develop an enhanced interest in sexuality, move toward self-sufficiency, and increase their competence and maturity.

There is a dynamic and interactive link between adolescents and their environments, and to make a successful transition to adulthood, adolescents must internalize societal norms that will enable them to develop self-esteem, establish and maintain social relationships, develop economic independence, form viable family units, and accept responsibility for self and others (Peterson, 1993; Zahn-Waxler, 1996). Adolescents must assume a variety of new roles, perform new tasks and activities, and participate in new environments. Research suggests that people vary in their abilities to establish role competencies and adapt to life situations (Hauser, Borman, Powers,

Jacobson, & Noam, 1990). The effects of changes during the developmental transition of adolescence can be long lasting (Peterson, 1993).

Social obstacles and social stigma play a dominant role during the adolescent period. Gray and Hahn (1997) defined *stigma* as "an undesirable difference that becomes a basis for separating an individual bearing such traits from the rest of society" (p. 395). Others impose stigma, and adolescents instinctively know and are acutely aware of any deviation in their appearance or traits that separate them from their peer group. For the adolescent, there is a constant struggle to reconcile reality with a desired image, and any dissonance can compromise self-image and self-esteem. Living with a disability intensifies the challenges adolescents confront in their efforts to adapt to social and cultural norms.

Issues for families and parents change as children progress through developmental periods, with adolescence marking a critical evolution in the roles of both child and parent: "Parents of children without disabilities experience relief from responsibility at this time; however, parents of children with disabilities, particularly those with severe disabilities, may feel the demands increase" (Case-Smith, 1991, p. 329). Relationships with parents and families are often strained during this phase of life for adolescents with special needs as they seek to overcome the isolation from their peers due to any stigma related to their activity limitations and participation restrictions. The family, whose physical and emotional resources may already be depleted or exhausted, often faces increased concern about the child's potential for isolation and vulnerability as he or she begins to move away from the familiar structures of the educational system to the community at large. Such concerns do not end when the child reaches adulthood; families of persons who have disabilities often continue to experience anxiety about future options for independent living and the aging and eventual death of the parents.

Adolescents must develop skills for basic and instrumental activities of daily living, education, work, leisure, and social participation to optimize their potential for a successful transition to the roles they will assume in their adult years. Because performance contexts—educational systems and workplaces—are so important to successful entry into adulthood, occupational therapy intervention can be targeted to these contexts to ensure that contexts are welcoming and accommodating. Education and work opportunities are dramatically reduced for people with physical, mental, and communication and interaction disabilities (McNeil, 1997). For some adolescents, the challenge is to match abilities with an appropriate vocational training, sheltered workshop, or community placement that will prepare them for and sustain them through adulthood.

The case studies of Barb and Alana in chapter 12 provide an opportunity for readers to use task analysis during evaluation and intervention with adolescent clients. The case study of Citizen Action Against Obesity in chapter 18 addresses the use of health promotion interventions and research evidence to combat the epidemic of obesity, an important population health issue.

Adult Occupations

Many cultures celebrate an individual's transition to adulthood because it represents the achievement of a state of maturity. For example, among North American cultures, many people celebrate their transition to adulthood through high school graduation ceremonies and proms. Although these occasions do not specifically acknowledge a "coming of age," they serve as a recognition of significant changes in life roles. Distinct events in the adult years mark transitions from adolescence to early, middle, and older adulthood. Adulthood as a phase of development begins with enhanced personal freedom, choice, and responsibility as one begins to separate from parents and siblings. It is a time of increased responsibility as one learns to care for oneself and others emotionally, spiritually, physically, and financially. In young adulthood one chooses a lifestyle and assumes new and complex roles: friend, lover, spouse, student, colleague, boss,

worker, breadwinner, volunteer, parent, and citizen, among others. The events considered most important at this stage are developing a vocational path to establish economic self-sufficiency, becoming a partner through cohabitation or marriage, and starting a family. One's identity as an adult is often shaped by the roles one assumes in society, and these roles are influenced by environmental and personal contexts. Indeed, competency as a worker is a primary social and cultural expectation of adults in most societies.

Adulthood can be turbulent yet stable, demanding yet straightforward, difficult yet rewarding. However, it is always a time of personal growth and transitions in performance patterns and lifestyles. Adults continue to experience physiological, psychological, and sociological changes after the transitions of young adulthood are over. Many of these changes reflect the societal roles of worker and provider, partner, parent, grandparent, and retiree (Hasselkus, 1998). During the middle years of adulthood, adults refine their vocational choices and skills through experience in the workforce and eventually anticipate and prepare for the transition to retirement. During these years social participation is crucial to role competency and adaptation as relationships are established and maintained with friends, lovers, spouses, partners, children, colleagues, neighbors, and others.

Although children and adolescents contribute to their communities, it is more common for adults to assume civic responsibilities and community leadership roles. Adults are paid workers, employers, organizational leaders, and volunteers. Adults hold responsibility for maintaining households, nurturing families, and building communities. Family units predominate in the social and cultural structure of society. *Family* is an operational term, not a categorical term; the family itself constitutes a complex and dynamic social unit (Donovan & McIntyre, 1985). For example, the sociocultural demand of Western societies on individuals to maintain highly productive career roles may become maladaptive as the family struggles to accommodate a plethora of roles and responsibilities that challenge value and belief systems around work and family roles and routines.

Traumatic injury or disease may interrupt adult roles, and persons challenged with resulting physical, mental, or communication and interaction disabilities must reestablish meaningful roles and patterns to resume engagement and participation. The case studies of Laurie, Jeff, and Rena in chapter 13 provide opportunities for readers to use task analysis in evaluation and intervention with adults adapting to new life circumstances. The case studies in chapter 16 describe workplace health promotion and injury prevention intervention strategies to address the needs of two populations of adults.

Older Adult Occupations

The roles that people assume change across the life span. Children become students when they enter school, adolescents become employees when they start their first job, adults become parents when they have their first child, and older adults become retirees when they leave the workforce. Just as other stages in the life span require individuals to adapt, so too does older adulthood. People are living longer than ever before, and society and everyday life are changing so rapidly that the process of aging is much different from that of the past. Older adults have been forced to create new guidelines on the "proper way to age" (Jackson, Mandel, Zemke, & Clark, 2001, p. 5).

Many older adults relinquish or experience a progressive loss of roles and occupations as they age. Indeed, older adults experience many life changes that place them at risk for social isolation and for loss of self-esteem and a sense of meaning to life. Changes in roles and performance patterns brought about by retirement and loss of spouses and friends can affect the breadth and depth of social participation. Conversely, occupations that older adults celebrate and that produce a sense of self-worth often seem mundane to others (e.g., going to movies, reading); these occupations are "salient occurrences in present life that often

embodied meaningful themes" from the perspective of older adults (Zemke & Clark, 1996, p. 358). The challenge to society and communities, therefore, is to find ways to enable older adults to age successfully. Continued engagement in daily activities provides meaning and temporal rhythm in life (Zemke & Clark, 1996).

Individuals differ in the ways they respond to growing old. This variability may be due to personal experiences, societal expectations of appropriate roles, cohort effects, or personality factors that influence attitudes toward aging, among other factors (Bonder, 1994). The personal capacities of older adults decrease at differential rates as well (Blau, 1973). "Aging brings 'typical' physical changes that may hamper a person's ability to actually perform day-to-day occupations" (Jackson et al., 2001, p. 5).

Increases in the population of older adults and in life expectancy have led to an increase in the prevalence of chronic disease. The population of older adults will continue to burgeon as the "baby boom" generation ages, suggesting that the size of the population with disabilities will increase in coming years. By the late 1990s, almost half of older adults had a disability, and one third had a severe disability (Bureau of the Census, 1997). This increase in the number of older people with disabilities is coinciding with a reduction in the availability of extended family; women, who in previous generations often acted as informal caregivers, are now largely in the workforce (Jackson et al., 2001).

Occupational therapy practitioners providing services to older adults who have or are at risk for activity limitations and participation restrictions can use task analysis to identify performance restrictions and limitations, activity demands, and contextual variables that limit engagement and to target intervention strategies at these barriers and risks. Services directed at enhancing older adults' access to daily activities within their community are consistent with the occupational therapy professional belief that older adults ought to be able to take part in the "naturally occurring activities of society" (AOTA, 1996, p. 855; Larson, Stevens-Ratchford, Pedretti, & Crabtree, 1996). The case studies of Nelson, Paul and Minnie, and Gladys and Gene in chapter 14 provide readers with opportunities to refine their skills in task analysis to address the needs of older clients and to consider health promotion and disability prevention strategies for the population of older people.

The Challenge

1. Track the trajectory of your life through infancy, preschool, school, and work. List the occupations at each stage that had primary and secondary influences on your life and development. Identify tasks and activities associated with these occupations. What prerequisite performance skills and patterns were required of you to enable you to engage in these occupations and participate in your customary contexts during each phase of development?

2. List tasks that were meaningful during your childhood because the "choice or control of the activity" was yours (Law, 2002a, p. 642). Consider when a lack of choice or control rendered a task less meaningful. Describe the value of engagement in meaningful tasks.

3. Consider the social and cultural contexts of your own adolescence. What social obstacles and cultural expectations had a significant positive or negative impact on you as an adolescent? Recall the impact of social and cultural contexts you have observed over time on peers who have a disability.

4. Discuss the social and cultural expectations that influence an adult's choice of work occupations. What social and cultural expectations influenced your decision to become an occupational therapy practitioner? Share this information with others who have chosen the same career path. Then describe the variability in social and cultural contexts that influenced this group of people.

5. Reflect on discussions you have previously had with an older adult about his or her occupational history. Consider the array of roles, occupations, tasks, and activities he or she engaged in over his or her life span. How might you structure an interview with an older client to establish an occupational profile during the evaluation phase of service delivery? How could this information be used during the course of intervention to ensure that occupational therapy services are meaningful? ■

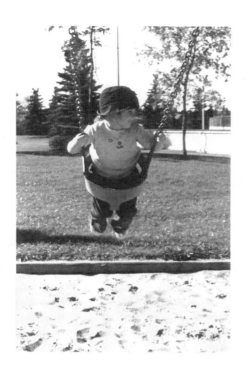

CHAPTER 7

Play as Occupation

Because we freely choose them, our play and leisure activities may be some of the purest expressions of who we are as a person.... If play is the purest expression of who we are as persons, then people who have lost their ability to play in the ways they choose have lost important pieces of themselves.

—Bundy, 1993, pp. 217, 220

CHAPTER OBJECTIVES
■ To describe the features, characteristics, and utility of purposeful play activities.
■ To describe the use of task analysis in defining the motor performance skills, sensory functions, and performance contexts that are challenged during participation in play.

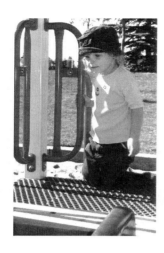

Play as Occupation

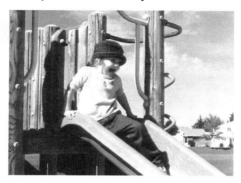

lay is internally controlled and intrinsically motivating. It focuses attention but suspends reality, stimulates behavior, requires participation, and allows freedom from externally imposed rules (Bundy, 1993). Play comprises both action and attitude, teaches symbolic meaning, leads to the pleasure of doing, and promotes skill acquisition (Ferland, 1992; Reilly, 1974). Playfulness is a way to approach activities, occupations, and circumstances. Indeed, play is a way to rehearse for life (Sabonis-Chafee & Hussey, 1998; Zemke & Clark, 1996).

Play is the primary occupation of children and is a precursor to the productive work habits, roles, and routines of adults (Reilly, 1974). A preschooler's imagination and imaginative play arise from and contribute to the development of autonomy and the quest for freedom to make decisions and take action. Young children develop initiative and gain a sense of independence when they begin to venture away from home to play in their neighborhoods. Children continue to develop a sense of identity and self-determination through adolescence when they select and engage in play, leisure, and other occupations (Shortridge, 1989). It is through playful experiences and engagement in play as an occupation that children develop and mature.

To foster engagement and participation in play, occupational therapy practitioners promote competency and facilitate adaptation by designing therapeutic activities, modifying activity demands, and altering environments. Practitioners, parents, and other caregivers can encourage a child to master challenges by supporting the different ways the child adapts to new tasks. Repetition and practice foster the child's confidence and self-esteem and promote greater success and satisfaction in engaging in occupations. Successful engagement, in turn, boosts the child's self-concept and confidence and supports his or her participation in contexts. Most pediatric intervention programs designed by occupational therapy practitioners aim, either directly or indirectly, to enable children to enhance their self-esteem (Mayberry, 1990; Willoughby, King, & Polatajko, 1996).

This chapter provides readers an opportunity to use task analysis to explore the impact of sensorimotor development on the occupation of play in the case study of Bobbie. For Bobbie to fully participate with his peers on the playground and engage in play occupations, he must develop several performance skills. Readers will establish an occupational profile and an analysis of Bobbie's occupational performance. Task analysis is the tool that will enable readers to evaluate perform-

CASE STUDY: BOBBIE

Bobbie is a 5-year-old boy who has just been assigned to your caseload following an evaluation by a registered occupational therapist at ABC Assessment Unit. Bobbie lives with his parents and sister in an apartment complex in a small town. He spends most weekends at his grandparents' farm and helps to care for their animals. Bobbie's father indicates that Bobbie is interested in dinosaurs, loves horses, and enjoys watching cartoons.

Bobbie's parents are worried about his confidence and self-esteem; he has a habit of withdrawing when he perceives that he cannot be successful. They are concerned about his lack of understanding of basic academic concepts, his inability to participate more fully in basic activities of daily living

(ADL), and his fear of playgrounds. Bobbie cannot identify letters, shapes, or colors, and he is unable to sort objects into same and different categories. He is unable to put on or remove his overcoat or manage his coat zipper and often places his shoes on the wrong feet. Bobbie is so afraid of the slide, swing set, and merry-go-round that he refuses to play on his own. Bobbie rides a tricycle short distances, but he cannot ride with the speed, agility, and precision of his friends. Some of his older friends have graduated to two-wheel bikes. Unfortunately, several children tease him because of his "clumsiness," and his parents are concerned that his fear of playgrounds limits his opportunities for social participation.

The occupational therapy report indicates that Bobbie's participation

in ADL, education, play, and leisure occupations is delayed in comparison to his peers. He has mild impairments in bilateral coordination, strength, and endurance and moderate impairments in trunk control, sequencing, and navigational skills. Sensory function testing also suggests mild impairments in proprioceptive, tactile, and vestibular function. ■

Learning Resources

Centre of Excellence for Early Childhood Development: www.excellence-earlychildhood.ca

Centres of Excellence for Children's Well-Being: www.hcsc.gc.ca/hppb/childhood-youth/centres/index2.html

National Institute of Child Health and Development: www.nichd.nih.gov

ance skills and patterns, contexts, activity demands, and client factors that affect Bobbie's participation in specific play tasks and activities. This information provides the foundation to plan a purposeful activity to challenge Bobbie's sensorimotor development, boost his confidence, and increase his self-esteem. The aim of intervention is to enhance Bobbie's engagement in the occupation of play.

Dimensions of Engagement and Participation

All of the dimensions of occupational performance influence a child's participation in the occupation of play: performance skills and patterns, contexts, activity demands, and client factors. Conversely, play provides a vehicle for the development of performance patterns as well as motor, process, communication, and interaction performance skills. This chapter focuses on the sensory body functions, motor performance skills,

and performance contexts that are challenged during participation in the occupation of play.

Sensory Body Functions and Motor Performance Skills

Participation in play contributes to the maturation and condition of body functions (i.e., client factors), and integrity of these functions enables children to participate in play. Participation in the play occupation promotes development, and because play promotes development, it can be used as an intervention. Occupational therapy practitioners who use play as a health intervention infuse play experiences, playfulness, and imaginative activities into the intervention process.

Through play and engagement in other occupations, children receive and process sensory information and produce motor responses. This requires both motor and process performance skills. The example of learning to ride a two-wheeled bike illustrates how sensory information and motor responses work together in developing a skill. Initially, children may be given training wheels to modify the demands of the activity. When they have gained confidence, those extra wheels are removed. To compensate for the greater difficulty and extra balance challenge, children typically sit on the seat and propel the bike with their feet on the ground. With practice, they can lift their feet and coast without falling. As their confidence increases, so does their willingness to try propelling with the pedals. As their postural stability and coordination improve, so do their chances for success. The self-confidence they gain through riding a bike prepares children to participate in neighborhood bicycle races and to venture long distances on errands. In this way, enhanced sensorimotor performance promotes children's engagement in community activities, social participation, and self-concept.

Sensory impairments affect people's ability to receive, process, and integrate incoming information. Perceptual impairments affect the ability to interpret this information, and motor impairments affect the production or expression of a desired response. Occupational therapy practitioners are trained in determining whether activity limitations are based on underlying sensory, perceptual, or motor functions. They use task analysis to evaluate the interaction of the child, his or her play tasks, and performance contexts and to design intervention that modifies activity demands or alters environments, or both, to facilitate a child's adaptation. Practitioners use remedial and restorative approaches to intervention to promote development or recovery of central nervous system functioning.

The *Occupational Therapy Practice Framework: Domain and Process* (American Occupational Therapy Association [AOTA], 2002) uses selected classifications from the *International Classification of Functioning, Disability and Health* (ICF) of the World Health Organization (WHO, 1980) to categorize sensory functions as seeing, hearing, vestibular, proprioceptive, and so forth. According to the *Framework,* motor performance skills are features of what one does or the observable elements of action that have implicit functional purposes (AOTA, 2002; Fisher & Kielhofner, 1995). More specifically, motor performance skills have five components, including (a) posture, (b) mobility, (c) coordination, (d) strength and effort, and (e) energy. The motor performance skills are defined in Appendix B, and sensory body functions are defined in Appendix F.

Performance Contexts

The performance contexts of children, including environmental factors (e.g., physical play areas, social context of day care) and personal factors (e.g., age, gender) must be considered in developing an occupational profile; they "represent the complete background of the individual's life and living" (WHO, 2001, p. 21). As they play, children both influence and are influenced by their environments.

The physical environment includes things such as accessibility and expectations for the function of the area (e.g., safe playground equipment and placement of furniture and activity centers). For the occupational therapy practitioner, the primary concern is "how physical settings shape naturally occurring activity and social interaction and with the symbolic meanings attached to places" (Spencer, 1998, p. 297).

Cultural, social, personal, spiritual, temporal, and virtual contextual factors (defined in Appendix D) all influence engagement in play. Culture and society place different developmental expectations on children of different ages, and the gender role expectations placed on boys and girls vary across sociocultural contexts. The socioeconomic status of persons and their communities is considered to be one of the most significant determinants of health (Evans, Barer, & Marmor, 1994; Ross et al., 2000; U.S. Department of Health and Human Services, 1998). This sociocultural contextual factor likely influences access to other important determinants of health, such as cohesive and nurturing communities, quality housing and play and leisure facilities, education and literacy, community resources, familial resources, economic opportunity, and so forth (Graham-Berman, Coupet, Egler, Mattis, & Banyard, 1996). A client's personal context includes his or her age, gender, socioeconomic status, and educational stage. Obviously, the chronological age of the child contributes to his or her ability to acquire motor and process performance skills. The *spiritual context* refers to the fundamental orientation of the child's life and includes whatever inspires or motivates him or her. *Spirit* represents the essence of the person and influences his or her selection of important occupations. *Temporal context* comes into play when stages of life, time of day, time of year, and so on are considered (AOTA, 2002). The *virtual context* refers to the communication environments that consist of such media as radio, television, and the Internet, in which persons communicate without physical contact. The virtual context of television has had a significant effect, both positive and negative, on child development (e.g., increased access to information and decreased physical activity).

Engagement and Participation in Play

As Ayres (1979) observed, "The interaction of the sensory and motor systems through all their countless interconnections is what gives meaning to sensation and purposefulness to movement.... Without interaction with the physical environment, learning is very difficult" (p. 46). Several evaluation methods are available for measuring the integrity of specific sensory, perceptual, and motor functions, but performance is used to determine the impact of impairments on engagement in occupation. It is through observation of clients' engagement in play and task analysis that occupational therapy practitioners create and test hypotheses regarding the performance skills, client factors, and activity demands that facilitate or hinder participation. Ayres described these sensory functions of learning to ride a bike as follows:

> Watch a child ride a bicycle and you will see how sensory stimulation leads to adaptive responses and adaptive responses lead to sensory integration. To balance himself and the bicycle, the child must sense the pull of gravity (vestibular) and the movements of his body (proprioception). Whenever he moves off center and begins to fall, his brain integrates the sensations of falling and forms an adaptive response. In this case, the adaptive response involves shifting the weight of the body to keep it balanced over the bicycle. If this adaptive response is not made, or is made too slowly, the child falls off the bicycle. If he repeatedly cannot make the adaptive response because he does not get good, precise information from his body and gravity senses, he may avoid riding a bicycle.
>
> Additional adaptive responses are needed to steer the bicycle so that it goes where the child wants it to go. To know where he and the bicycle are in relation to a tree, his brain must integrate visual sensations with body sensations and the pull of gravity. Then it must use those sensations to plan a path around the tree. The faster the bicycle goes, the greater the sensory stimulation and the more accurate the adaptive response must be. If the child rides into a tree, it means that his brain did not integrate the sensations, or it did not do so quickly enough. When a child gets off his bicycle after a successful ride, his brain knows more about gravity and the space around his body and how his body moves, and so riding a bicycle becomes easier each time. This is how sensory integration develops. (pp. 14–15)[1]

The Challenge

1. Review and refamiliarize yourself with Figure 3.2 and the definitions of terms from the *Occupational Therapy Practice Framework: Domain and Process* in the areas of motor performance skills (Appendix B), context (Appendix D), and sensory functions (Appendix F).

[1]From *Sensory Integration and the Child* © 1979 by Western Psychological Services. Reprinted with permission of the publisher, Western Psychological Services, 12031 Wilshire Boulevard, Los Angeles, CA 90025 U.S.A. Not to be reprinted in whole or in part for any additional purpose without the expressed, written permission of the publisher. All rights reserved.

2. What gross motor play and leisure activities did you participate in and enjoy during early childhood? What are the characteristics and qualities of these activities that influenced the activity demands required of you? Activity demands are the aspects of an activity (e.g., required equipment and space, process used to carry out the activity, required actions) and the required underlying body functions and structures needed to carry out the activity. Activity demands are defined in Appendix E.

3. Read "Position Paper: Purposeful Activity" (AOTA, 1993) (Appendix L). What are the features or characteristics of a purposeful activity? Does the occupation of play qualify as a purposeful activity? Is riding a tricycle a purposeful activity? Reflect on how riding a tricycle enhanced your performance skills and the functional integrity of your client factors during your childhood. How did riding a tricycle allow you to participate in your play occupations?

4. Read the case study of Bobbie and review the abridged version of the Client Profile and Task Analysis Form in Figure 7.1, which has been partially completed. Work toward completing this form by summarizing the activity demands of playing on a slide, swing set, and merry-go-round and riding a tricycle with speed, agility, and precision. This abridged version includes subsections of the full form that reflect the focus of this chapter: motor skills, sensory functions, and contexts. (The full Client Profile and Task Analysis Form is provided in Appendix J.)

5. Profile Bobbie's performance patterns and rate his motor performance skills using the qualifiers listed in the appropriate section of Figure 7.1. Use the information available in the case study to profile Bobbie's abilities and the extent of any impairments in his sensory functions using the following qualifiers: 0 (no impairment), 1 (mild impairment), 2 (moderate impairment), 3 (severe impairment), 4 (complete impairment), 8 (not specified),

and 9 (not applicable). This impairment scale is used in the ICF system (WHO, 2001). If you wish to profile other motor performance skills and client factors, use a complete version of the Client Profile and Task Analysis Form (Appendix J).

6. Rate the level of challenge of each activity demand and compare these ratings to ratings of Bobbie's sensory functions. Use the following ICF activity demand qualifiers to rate the degree of challenge to each sensory function: 1 (mild challenge), 2 (moderate challenge), 3 (maximum challenge), and 9 (not applicable).

To complete the analysis of Bobbie's motor performance skills and sensory functions, answer the following questions. Notice that you will be creating and, over the course of therapy, will have the opportunity to test hypotheses regarding the performance skills, activity demands, and client factors that support or hinder Bobbie's participation in play.

a. Why do you think Bobbie is fearful of the slide, swing, and merry-go-round? What motor performance skills are required for success on these three pieces of equipment (i.e., activity demands)? Does the case study indicate that Bobbie has activity limitations in these dimensions? Does he have impairments in sensory functions that might compromise the development of these performance skill competencies?

b. Why do you think Bobbie has difficulty riding his tricycle with "speed, agility, and precision"? What motor performance skills are required to ride a tricycle in this manner? Does the case study indicate that Bobbie has difficulty with these performance skills as a result of sensory impairments?

c. Why do you think Bobbie is unable to put on or remove his overcoat, manage his zipper, and place his shoes on the proper feet? What motor skills are required to complete these activities? Does the case study indicate that Bobbie has difficulty in these per-

CLIENT PROFILE AND TASK ANALYSIS FORM

CLIENT PROFILE

Name: *Bobbie*

Occupational history: *Lives in an apartment complex in a small town, spends a lot of time at grandparents' farm, and helps to care for their animals*

Patterns of daily living (see also performance patterns):

Interests, values, and needs: *Interest in dinosaurs and enjoys horses and cartoons. Fear of playgrounds. Parents are worried about confidence and self-esteem, and they are concerned about Bobbie's fear of the playground and lack of understanding of academic concepts.*

TASK ANALYSIS

Task: *Playing on the slide, swing set, and merry-go-round*
Riding a tricycle with speed, agility, and precision

ACTIVITY DEMANDS

Objects used: *Slide, swing set, merry-go-round, tricycle and two-wheel bike*

Space demands: *Playground with equipment, safe location to ride*

Social demands: *Can do the task alone or with one or more people*

Sequence and timing:

Required actions:
1.
2.
3.
4.
5.
6.
7.
8.
9.
10.
See Activity Demands and Client Factors section of this form for required body functions and structures.

AREAS OF OCCUPATION

Check the area or areas that apply.		Relevance and meaning for client:
Activities of daily living (ADL)	☐	_____
Instrumental ADL	☐	_____
Education	☐	_____
Work	☐	_____
Play	☐	_____
Leisure	☐	_____
Social participation	☐	_____

PERFORMANCE PATTERNS

Habits: *Withdraws from challenges when he perceives that he will not be successful*

Routines: *Goes to farm every week*

Roles: *Son, day care student, brother*

Continued

Figure 7.1. Client Profile and Task Analysis Form: Abridged and partially completed for the case study of Bobbie.

PERFORMANCE SKILLS

Qualifiers: 0 (no impairment), 1 (mild impairment), 2 (moderate impairment), 3 (severe impairment),
4 (complete impairment), 8 (not specified), 9 (not applicable)

Motor skills		Qualifier	*Motor skills*		Qualifier
Posture:	Stabilizes	☐	Strength and effort:	Moves	☐
	Aligns	☐		Transports	☐
	Positions	☐		Lifts	☐
Mobility:	Walks	☐		Calibrates	☐
	Reaches	☐		Grips	☐
	Bends	☐	Energy:	Endures	☐
Coordination:	Coordinates	☐		Paces	☐
	Manipulates	☐			
	Flows	☐			

Comments:

ACTIVITY DEMANDS AND CLIENT FACTORS

Activity demand qualifiers
Level of challenge required to perform:
1 (mild challenge), 2 (moderate challenge),
3 (maximum challenge), 9 (not applicable)

Client factor qualifiers
Level of client impairment: 0 (no impairment), 1 (mild impairment), 2 (moderate impairment), 3 (severe impairment), 4 (complete impairment), 8 (not specified), 9 (not applicable)

Level of Demand
Comments and qualifier:

		Sensory functions and pain		**Level of Impairment** *Qualifier and comments:*
_____	☐	Seeing functions	☐	_____
_____	☐	Hearing function	☐	_____
_____	☐	Vestibular function	☐	_____
_____	☐	Taste and smell functions	☐	_____
_____	☐	Proprioceptive function	☐	_____
_____	☐	Touch functions	☐	_____
_____	☐	Sensory functions related to temperature and other stimuli	☐	_____
_____	☐	Sensations of pain	☐	_____

CONTEXTS

External to the client
Cultural context (e.g., laws, resources, opportunities):

Physical context:

Social context:

Temporal context (e.g., time of day, year):

Virtual context:

Internal to the client
Personal context:

Spiritual context:

Cultural context (e.g., customs, values, beliefs):

Temporal context (e.g., age, stage of life):

Figure 7.1. Client Profile and Task Analysis Form: Abridged and partially completed for the case study of Bobbie *(continued).*

formance skills due to sensory impairments pertinent to these performance skills?

7. Use the information you have compiled to list Bobbie's client goals in Table 7.1, which has been started for you. A suggested format for writing goals is provided in Appendix K. Ensure that the goals are written in such a way that they both communicate the intent to maintain or promote performance and prevent dysfunction and fit the concerns, priorities, and resources of the family. In the clinical setting, you would establish these goals in collaboration with Bobbie's parents.

Long-term goals define target outcomes in occupational performance areas (AOTA, 1994a). Short-term objectives relate to the skills and patterns that are small units of performance, impairments and client factors that must be addressed, or the activity or environmental domains that require change if the long-term goal is to be achieved. Goals must be specific, objective, and measurable.

8. During the latest intervention session, the occupational therapy practitioner used therapeutic use of self to create a playful and imaginative context in which to facilitate Bobbie's development in the areas specified in Goals 1 and 3 (see Table 7.1). Bobbie participated in a purposeful activity. The practitioner worked with Bobbie to select and design an obstacle course using a farm theme because Bobbie's visits to his grandfather's farm were a meaningful occupation to him. The obstacle course was designed to augment Bobbie's confidence and performance skills on the playground. Bobbie cut out a yellow paper star (sheriff's badge), wore a weighted vest (cowboy jacket) to walk across a balance beam (barnyard fence), threw red and blue beanbags (hay bales) into separate baskets, and bounced on a small trampoline (horse). Considering the therapeutic activity designed for Bobbie, ask yourself these questions:

a. Why was Bobbie asked to cut out a paper star? What are the activity demands?

Table 7.1. Client goals for Bobbie.

Short-Term Goal	Long-Term Objectives
1. Bobbie will independently play on a swing set and slide for 3 minutes with confidence.	1a. Bobbie will improve his vestibular and proprioceptive processing, trunk control, and bilateral coordination to climb the ladder of the slide independently by the end of the school year. 1b. Bobbie will increase his confidence with vestibular movement by first using a toddler swing seat, then progressing to an open sling seat within 2 months with daily play opportunities.
2. Bobbie will develop his understanding of academic concepts of color and numbers from early preschool levels to a 4-year-old level by the end of the school year.	2a. Bobbie will separate red and blue objects into color categories during activity time at school and generalize this skill across activities by the next school term. 2b.
3. Bobbie will ride his tricycle through an obstacle course with improved speed and agility as demonstrated by ease of performance and increased participation within 6 weeks with daily opportunity to practice.	3a. 3b.
4.	4a. 4b.

b. Why did Bobbie wear a weighted vest? How does this relate to the client factors noted in the case study and the challenge of the task?

c. What activity demands are challenges for Bobbie when he walks across the balance beam, sorts and throws beanbags, and bounces on a trampoline?

d. How could academic skills be incorporated into this activity so that learning occurs in a fun context?

9. Reconstruct and perform this obstacle course. Assume that Bobbie has mastered this activity. How could you increase the activity demands to enhance the challenge and continue to develop Bobbie's motor skills and sensory functions?

10. Design and construct an additional activity for Bobbie to do while engaging in this obstacle course. The activity should challenge and promote the development of areas identified in the short-term objectives. Use balls, mats, balance beams, barrels, beanbags, hoops, foam blocks, swings, and any other available objects. Be sure to create a meaningful context for this play activity.

11. Bobbie has mastered this new activity. Continue to provide Bobbie with a challenge that is achievable by altering the activity to make it slightly more difficult. Explain why purposeful activities should balance achievement with challenge.

12. Take turns role-playing as Bobbie and his occupational therapy practitioner with another person. Explore the different frames of reference (e.g., sensory integration) a practitioner might use to guide practice. Role-playing will increase the accuracy of your task and activity analysis and enable you to practice interacting with a young child. The verbal and nonverbal interactive relationship between therapist and client provides encouragement, motivation, and feedback to reinforce and facilitate learning.

13. How might a community support the occupation of play and the subsequent developmental benefits that accrue to children who have play-based experiences? Consider how a community could influence activities in day care centers, preschool programs, and schools. How might a community get together to collaboratively define goals, objectives, and an implementation plan to contribute to a healthy future for children? ■

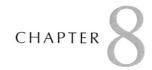

CHAPTER 8

Education as Occupation

Childhood is hopeful and joyful and ever new.
The spirit, the playfulness, and joy of childhood creates the
context for occupational therapy for children.

—Case-Smith, Allen, & Pratt, 1996, p. 3

CHAPTER OBJECTIVES
- To describe how occupational therapy practitioners apply task analysis as an evaluation and intervention tool to develop intervention strategies that enable young clients to participate in the occupation of education.
- To define performance patterns, process performance skills, communication and interaction performance skills, and mental functions as these dimensions relate to the occupation of education.
- To apply task analysis to profile the performance patterns, performance skills, and mental functions that are challenged during participation in educational activities.

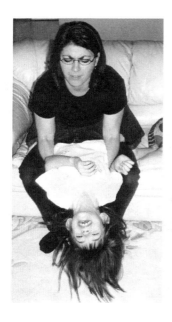

Education as Occupation

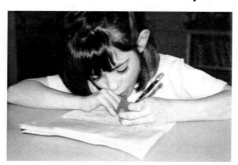

By the time children enter school, they typically have grown accustomed to a high level of activity through the occupation of play as infants, toddlers, and preschoolers. Once children take on the role of student, they are expected to adapt to new rules of classroom and playground conduct and to make the transition between these two environmental contexts quickly. As children change contexts and mature, they experience a decline in physical activity; less time is available for play because teachers place increasing emphasis on directing children's energy and attention span toward the education occupation. Children's abilities to endure and pace academic tasks are nurtured, and they are guided in establishing more formal daily routines and habits. Children perform several of tasks each day while engaging in their student role. They also establish new performance patterns (e.g., daily routines) by virtue of a scheduled school day, week, and year (i.e., temporal contexts).

Although the education occupation occupies many hours in the life of a child, the importance of the student role and academic achievement varies among children, families, and cultures. Children's interests, values, and needs, as well as their personal and environmental contexts, shape

the meaning and purpose they attribute to different educational activities. In essence, the meaningfulness of an activity depends on a personal interpretation of its value or importance. Thus, the initial step of the occupational therapy process involves creating an occupational profile that captures the essence of the child's occupational history, interests, values, performance patterns, and personal context. Then, practitioners conduct a broader analysis of the child's occupations, performance, and contexts.

This chapter provides readers an opportunity to use task analysis to increase their understanding of a child's participation in education through the case study of Tina. Readers will establish an occupational profile and an analysis of Tina's performance to identify her interests, values, and needs, as well as the performance patterns and skills, contexts, and client factors that affect her participation. This profile provides the foundation to plan a purposeful activity to challenge her sensorimotor and cognitive functions and to teach others how to structure and use therapeutic activities to promote performance skills and engagement in the education occupation. Readers will complete long-term and short-term goals that address Tina's performance skills and patterns, client factors, and

CASE STUDY: TINA

Tina will be turning 6 years old next month and has already started to talk about her upcoming birthday party at ABC Day Care and Kindergarten. The child care workers and teachers at ABC are very fond of Tina; they have taken care of her weekdays since she was 9 months old. Tina is an only child and lives with her father. ABC's case manager requests an occupational therapy consultation and explains Tina's situation.

According to her case manager, Tina has always been a very active child. "Although she is very uncoordinated for her age, she loves gross-motor activities and is usually a 'daredevil' on the playground. Her social skills are quite immature. She likes to play in the same area as other children, but does not play with them in a cooperative or collaborative fash-

ion. She listens well, but doesn't seem to ask for things when she needs or wants them and must be encouraged to do this." Over the past year or so, the case manager has become increasingly concerned about Tina's short attention span and lack of interest in tabletop or quiet-time activities. She has great difficulty completing puzzles and becomes frustrated when trying to use scissors. She can cut a straight line, but the teacher has to explain how to turn the paper to cut around shapes. Tina loves to color pictures but is not very good at it. Although she puts great effort into printing, Tina cannot print letters in sequence to spell her name.

After spending a half hour interviewing some of the staff members, you realize that ABC provides a very unstructured approach to learning. Children are encouraged to pursue

activities of interest to themselves. Although the teachers offer projects that facilitate learning, the students can choose not to participate.

After Tina's evaluation is complete, you determine that she has poor fine-motor coordination and a very immature pencil grasp and has not yet established hand dominance. Her temporal and spatial organization, visuospatial perception, and sequencing skills are also below average. Tina appears to be very self-conscious about her verbal skills and about her performance when completing puzzles and paper-and-pencil activities. She loves animals, the circus, and gymnastics. ◾

Learning Resource

U.S. Department of Education, Office of Special Education and Rehabilitation Services: www.ed.gov/offices/OSERS/

---

contexts. Role competence is one of the occupational therapy outcomes identified in the Occupational Therapy Service Model (see Figure 1.1) and reflects clients' ability to effectively meet the demands of roles in which they elect to engage (American Occupational Therapy Association [AOTA], 2002).

Dimensions of Engagement and Participation

All of the dimensions of occupational performance influence a person's participation in the education occupation: performance skills and patterns, contexts, activity demands, and client factors. This chapter focuses on performance patterns, mental functions, and performance skills that are challenged during participation in the occupation of education.

Performance Patterns

The *Occupational Therapy Practice Framework: Domain and Process* (AOTA, 2002) defines *performance patterns* as client's roles, routines, and habits. *Roles* are "a set of behaviors that have some socially agreed upon function and for which there is an accepted code of norms" (Christiansen & Baum, 1997, p. 603). Certain behaviors or roles are expected of students. *Routines* are activities that have established sequences, whereas *habits* are those "automatic behaviours that are integrated into more complex patterns that enable people to function on a day-to-day basis" (Neistadt & Crepeau, 1998a, p. 869). Habits either support or interfere with performance, and they can be categorized as useful, impoverished, or dominating (AOTA, 2002). Appendix C defines performance patterns of concern to occupational therapy practitioners.

Mental Functions

Conformity to the student role is often measured in the classroom by evaluation of a child's energy, attention span, and temperament. Academic performance is often rated primarily on the basis of success at tasks requiring mental functions and cognition. Mental functions include affective, cognitive, and perceptual abilities (AOTA, 2002). The affective (i.e., feeling) domain comprises all social and emotional functions and includes both interpersonal and intrapersonal dimensions. The cognitive (i.e., thinking) domain comprises all mental functions, both cognitive and intellectual, including comprehension, judgment, and reasoning (Canadian Association of Occupational Therapists [CAOT], 1997). The term *cognition* is frequently used in practice to refer to the mental functions required for the process skills of acquiring and using knowledge, thinking, and performing higher brain functions, as well as processing, storing, retrieving, and manipulating information (AOTA, 1994b; Quintana, 1995). The term *perception* is used in practice to refer to the process of interpreting sensory stimuli (e.g., tactile, visual, auditory) and visuospatial information.

The *Occupational Therapy Practice Framework* (AOTA, 2002) categorizes mental functions as global or specific. *Global mental functions* include such dimensions as temperament, personality, energy, and drive. *Specific mental functions* include attention, memory, perception, thought, higher-level cognitive functions, language, and emotional regulation (AOTA, 2002). Mental functions, together with other client factors, provide the foundation for the development of performance skills. Appendix F defines the client factors of concern to occupational therapy practitioners.

Performance Skills

The education occupation and student role require motor, process, and communication and interaction performance skills. For example, when children begin school, they are expected to learn to initiate, sequence, and terminate activities (i.e.,

process skills); grasp and manipulate crayons and pencils (i.e., motor skills); and engage and collaborate with others (i.e., communication and interaction skills). The different types of performance skills interact among themselves and with the mental functions.

According to the *Occupational Therapy Practice Framework, process performance skills* include skills "used in managing and modifying actions on route to the completion of daily life tasks" (Fisher & Kielhofner, 1995, p. 120). There are five categories of process skills: (a) sustaining effort over the course of a task; (b) seeking and using task-related knowledge; (c) organizing temporal information pertaining to the beginning, logical ordering, continuation, and completion of the steps and action sequences of a task; (d) organizing space and objects; and (e) adapting to immutable circumstances (AOTA, 2002). Appendix B defines performance skills of concern to occupational therapy practitioners.

Communication and interaction performance skills are those skills required to convey intentions and needs and coordinate social behavior to act together with people (Forsyth & Kielhofner, 1999; Forsyth, Salamy, Simon, & Kielhofner, 1997). There are three categories of communication and interaction skills: (a) physicality, or use of the physical body when communicating, including physical contact, gaze, gestures, maneuvers, orientation of body in relation to others, and postures; (b) information exchange, which involves articulation, assertion, asking, engaging, expression, modulation, sharing, speaking, and sustaining speech for appropriate duration; and (c) relations with others, including collaboration, conformity, focus, relationship and rapport, and respect (AOTA, 2002). Appendix B defines performance skills of concern to occupational therapy practitioners.

People possess attributes, skills, and abilities that make them unique as individuals and enable them to process emotions and interact with family, peers, and others in their community. Communication and interaction performance skills require or are dependent on mental functions such as language and emotional functions (CAOT, 1997). When children enter school, they rapidly expand their circle of friends and acquaintances and the size of their social network. Therefore, the student role requires development and refinement of communication and interaction skills beyond the toddler level.

Teachers learn about the mental functions of students through the actions and words children use to communicate, and these performance skills serve as one of the primary measures of academic achievement. Examples of abilities that teachers look for in the early years to assess the maturity of mental functions include the abilities to recognize shapes, sizes, and objects; to sort and categorize information and objects; and to generalize concepts. The ability to understand language and express oneself through speech is vital to the interactive process of learning and the measurement of the outcome of knowledge acquisition.

As the student matures, performance skills in the area of written communication develop; mental and motor functions are refined to enable students to print and cursive write. For example, a mature tripod grasp supports acquisition of those graphic skills (see Figure 8.1). Perceptual functions required for written communication are interrelated with the concurrent development of visuospatial perception and memory functions, as well as the sensory integration of tactile, proprioceptive, and visual stimuli. Written communication, in the

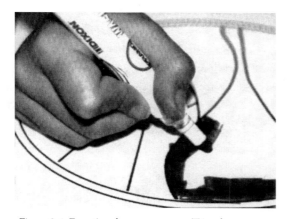

Figure 8.1. Functional grasp patterns: Tripod grasp.

form of either paper-and-pencil or computer-generated documents, is the principal way that children demonstrate their acquisition of higher-level cognitive functions such as concept formation and problem solving. As students progress in school, measurement of academic achievement is increasingly based on written communication. Children's sense of competency in school is based in turn on their academic achievement and their identity as a student who does school work.

Engagement and Participation in School

The majority of elementary school class time is spent on paper-and-pencil and manipulative tasks, a problem for the majority of children with learning difficulties who demonstrate fine-motor and handwriting difficulties (McHale & Cermak, 1992). In work with preschoolers and young students with learning disabilities or motor performance delays, occupational therapy practitioners evaluate the client factors required to perform functional classroom activities and then use strategies and techniques to improve these skills (Case-Smith et al., 1996).

Occupational therapy practitioners, who understand engagement from a holistic perspective, must address all aspects of performance when providing intervention designed to support engagement in occupations (AOTA, 2002). Student clients can be individual children, groups of children, or an entire population of students. Practitioners work toward enabling these clients to engage in the education occupation in varied classroom contexts by enhancing performance patterns, performance skills, and client factors and by altering activity demands and promoting enabling school contexts.

Occupational therapy services can also prepare children to adjust to residual activity limitations following trauma, disorder, or disease. In work with children with mental function impairments and cognitive disabilities in academic contexts, for example, practitioners direct intervention toward providing purposeful activities to enhance performance patterns and skills (i.e., remediation or restoration), altering activity demands, and restructuring performance contexts to compensate for mental function impairments (i.e., compensation or adaptation). Occupational therapy intervention can also be directed toward providing opportunities for students to practice new methods (i.e., compensation or adaptation), training and consulting with teachers and parents to create an enriched context for all children (i.e., health promotion), and reducing the occurrence of barriers to optimal participation (i.e., disability prevention).

When selecting therapeutic activities to challenge a particular child's abilities and promote more advanced performance skills, the practitioner directs initial intervention at lower-order performance processes such as orientation and attention (Abreu & Toglia, 1987). Elements that can be graded to enhance the therapeutic value of an activity include environmental structure, activity familiarity, directions for completion, number of items, spatial arrangement of items, and response rate required (Wheatley, 1996). Purposeful and meaningful activity is the foundation for motivation (Hess & Campion, 1983; Kirscher, 1984; Trombly, 1995a); personal satisfaction (Thibodeaux & Ludwig, 1988); learning and adaptation (Yuen, 1988); and motor skills development and performance (Hsieh, Nelson, Smith, & Peterson, 1996; Licht & Nelson, 1990; Yuen, 1988).

To design effective and efficient evaluation and intervention, occupational therapy practitioners partner with parents, teachers, and others to identify educational goals that are important to a student and his or her family (or a group of students and their families). An individual student's educational goals are documented by the occupational therapy practitioner as part of an educational team's contribution to an individualized education program. Communication is vital to the process of goal setting; the process of sharing their interests, needs, values, and priorities is vital to a client's sense of autonomy in directing his or her own services. Parents, teachers, and other stakeholders may act as proxies for children by providing information regarding the activities that have meaning and purpose to the child.

The Challenge

1. Review and refamiliarize yourself with the definition of terms from the *Occupational Therapy Practice Framework* in the areas of performance skills (Appendix B), performance patterns (Appendix C), and client factors such as mental functions (Appendix F).

2. From the suggestions below, select and perform one activity that a child might engage in at school. What process skills, communication and interaction performance skills, and mental functions are used during participation in the educational activity you selected?
   Preschool level: Place a circle, square, and triangle into a form board. Color a picture. Play Simon Says.
   Elementary level: Use a pattern to construct a three-dimensional object. Draw a clock that tells the current time. Build a fort. Print the letters of the alphabet. Tie shoelaces.
      Review Figure 3.2 and the activity demands defined in the *Occupational Therapy Practice Framework* (Appendix E). Use Figure 8.2 to rate the degree of challenge to each type of mental function required for the activity you selected.

3. Read the case study of Tina and review the abridged Client Profile and Task Analysis Form in Figure 8.3. Work toward completing this form by profiling the activity demands of completing puzzles, using scissors, and spelling a name. Figure 8.3 includes subsections of the full form that reflect the focus of this chapter: performance patterns, mental functions, and performance skills. (The full Client Profile and Task Analysis form is provided in Appendix J.)

4. Using the information in the case study, profile Tina's performance patterns and process and her communication and interaction performance skills in Figure 8.3. Also profile her abilities and impairments in mental functioning.

ACTIVITY DEMANDS AND CLIENT FACTORS

Activity demand qualifiers

Level of challenge required to perform: 1 (mild challenge), 2 (moderate challenge), 3 (maximum challenge), 9 (not applicable)

Comments	Qualifier	Body Functions
		Mental Functions: Global
_____	☐	Consciousness functions
_____	☐	Orientation functions
_____	☐	Sleep
_____	☐	Temperament and personality functions
_____	☐	Energy and drive functions
		Mental Functions: Specific
_____	☐	Attention functions
_____	☐	Memory functions
_____	☐	Perceptual functions
_____	☐	Thought functions
_____	☐	Higher-level cognitive functions
_____	☐	Mental functions of language
_____	☐	Calculation functions
_____	☐	Mental functions of sequencing complex movement
_____	☐	Psychomotor functions
_____	☐	Emotional functions
_____	☐	Experience of self and time functions

Figure 8.2. Activity demands: Required mental functions.

5. What mental functions are required for completing puzzles, using scissors, and spelling a name? List Tina's abilities, and rate her limitations in Figure 8.3.

6. To complete the analysis of process and communication and interaction performance skills and mental functions, answer the following questions. Notice that you will be creating and, over the course of the intervention, will have the opportunity to test hypotheses regarding the performance skills, activity demands, and client factors that support or hinder Tina's participation in play.

   a. Why do you think Tina has difficulty completing puzzles, using scissors, and spelling her name? What process performance skills and mental functions are required for successful participation in these activities? Does the case study indicate that Tina has difficulty with these performance skills? Does she have impairments in mental functions pertinent to these performance skills?

   b. Why do you think Tina "likes to play in the same area as other children, but does not play with them in a cooperative or collaborative fashion" and "listens well, but doesn't seem to ask for things when she needs or wants them and must be encouraged to do this"? What communication and interaction performance skills are required for more age-appropriate social skills?

   c. The case manager indicates that Tina is a very active child but is concerned about her short attention span and lack of interest in tabletop or quiet-time activities. How do temporal contextual factors, such as chronological and developmental age, and the social and cultural contextual factors at ABC Day Care and Kindergarten affect Tina and her role performance patterns?

   d. What process performance skills does Tina need to support her engagement in school activities in which she is expected to participate?

CLIENT PROFILE AND TASK ANALYSIS FORM

CLIENT PROFILE

Name: *Tina*

Occupational history:

Patterns of daily living (see also performance patterns):

Interests, values, and needs:

TASK ANALYSIS

Task:

ACTIVITY DEMANDS

Objects used:

Space demands:

Social demands:

Sequence and timing:

Required actions:
1.
2.
3.
4.
5.
6.
7.
8.
9.
10.

AREAS OF OCCUPATION

Check the area or areas that apply.   *Relevance and meaning for client:*

Activities of daily living (ADL)   ☐   _____
Instrumental ADL   ☐   _____
Education   ☐   _____
Work   ☐   _____
Play   ☐   _____
Leisure   ☐   _____
Social participation   ☐   _____

PERFORMANCE PATTERNS

Habits:

Routines:

Roles:

Continued

Figure 8.3. Client Profile and Task Analysis Form: Abridged for the case study of Tina.

PERFORMANCE SKILLS

Qualifiers: 0 (no impairment), 1 (mild impairment), 2 (moderate impairment), 3 (severe impairment), 4 (complete impairment), 8 (not specified), 9 (not applicable)

Process Skills		Qualifier	*Communication and Interaction Skills*		Qualifier
Energy:	Paces	☐	Physicality:	Contacts	☐
	Attends	☐		Gazes	☐
Knowledge:	Chooses	☐		Gestures	☐
	Uses	☐		Maneuvers	☐
	Handles	☐		Orients	☐
	Heeds	☐		Postures	☐
	Inquires	☐	Relations:	Collaborates	☐
Temporal				Conforms	☐
organization:	Initiates	☐		Focuses	☐
	Continues	☐		Relates	☐
	Sequences	☐		Respects	☐
	Terminates	☐	Information exchange:	Articulates	☐
Organization of space				Asserts	☐
and objects:	Searches or locates	☐		Asks	☐
	Gathers	☐		Engages	☐
	Organizes	☐		Expresses	☐
	Restores	☐		Modulates	☐
	Navigates	☐		Shares	☐
Adaptation:	Notices or responds	☐		Speaks	☐
	Accommodates	☐		Sustains	☐
	Adjusts	☐	Comments:		
	Benefits	☐			

Comments:

ACTIVITY DEMANDS AND CLIENT FACTORS

Activity demand qualifiers

Level of challenge required to perform:
1 (mild challenge), 2 (moderate challenge),
3 (maximum challenge), 9 (not applicable)

Client factor qualifiers

Level of client impairment: 0 (no impairment), 1 (mild impairment), 2 (moderate impairment), 3 (severe impairment), 4 (complete impairment), 8 (not specified), 9 (not applicable)

Level of Demand	**Body Functions**	**Level of Impairment**
Comments and qualifier:		*Qualifier and comments:*
	Mental functions: Global	
_____ ☐	Consciousness functions	☐ _____
_____ ☐	Orientation functions	☐ _____
_____ ☐	Sleep	☐ _____
_____ ☐	Temperament and personality functions	☐ _____
_____ ☐	Energy and drive functions	☐ _____
	Mental functions: Specific	
_____ ☐	Attention functions	☐ _____
_____ ☐	Memory functions	☐ _____
_____ ☐	Perceptual functions	☐ _____
_____ ☐	Thought functions	☐ _____
_____ ☐	Higher-level cognitive functions	☐ _____
_____ ☐	Mental functions of language	☐ _____
_____ ☐	Calculation functions	☐ _____
_____ ☐	Mental functions of sequencing complex movement	☐ _____
_____ ☐	Psychomotor functions	☐ _____
_____ ☐	Emotional functions	☐ _____
_____ ☐	Experience of self and time functions	☐ _____

Continued

Figure 8.3. Client Profile and Task Analysis Form: Abridged for the case study of Tina *(continued).*

CONTEXTS

External to the client	*Internal to the client*
Cultural context (e.g., laws, resources, opportunities):	Personal context:
Physical context:	Spiritual context:
Social context:	Cultural context (e.g., customs, values, beliefs):
Temporal context (e.g., time of day, year):	Temporal context (e.g., age, stage of life):
Virtual context:	

Figure 8.3. Client Profile and Task Analysis Form: Abridged for the case study of Tina *(continued).*

7. Use the information you have compiled to list Tina's client goals in Table 8.1, which has been started for you. Ensure that the goals fit the concerns, priorities, and resources of this family and day care center. In the clinical setting, you would establish these goals on behalf of Tina in collaboration with her father, the teacher, and any other special education professionals and staff at ABC Day Care and Kindergarten. A suggested format for writing client goals and information regarding how to complete this form are provided in Appendix K.

8. During the first intervention session, Tina participated in a therapeutic activity that the occupational therapy practitioner developed for the class. The activity allowed the children a degree of movement around the classroom to seek supplies and facilitated a positive outcome on a paper-and-pencil craft activity to be a gift for the children's parents. The project

Table 8.1. Client goals for Tina.

Long-Term Goal	Short-Term Objectives
1. Tina will print her name by forming letters in the correct sequence	1a. Tina will trace the letters in her name to learn the required motor plan. 1b. Tina will sequence the letters in her name by copying from a template on her first try, then print her name without cues immediately afterward.
2.	2a. 2b.
3.	3a. 3b.
4.	4a. 4b.

required the children to find a shape or object in the room to represent the center of a sunflower and then trace it onto a piece of construction paper. Tina found a can of the right size and successfully traced around the bottom of the can to make a circle. The next step was to go outside with a partner and find leaves or flower petals to paste around the circle as petals. Once Tina and her partner were back at the table, the practitioner asked them to tell others about the shapes and colors they found. Tina then glued the petals onto the paper. She shredded tissue paper and glued it into the center of the flower. The occupational therapy practitioner held the stems in his hand and waited for the children to ask him to pass them a stem. Tina stood at the table to perform this craft.

a. Why was the activity designed to include structured movement?

b. Why was Tina asked to trace around an object? What are the activity demands?

c. Why did Tina shred rather than cut the paper to decorate the center of the sunflower?

d. How do the strategies relate to noted client factors and the challenge of the task?

e. What are the activity demands of locating an object, tracing it, collecting leaves, shredding paper, and gluing everything together?

f. What communication and interaction performance skills were required? What strategies might be used to enhance communication among the students?

g. Assume that Tina has mastered this activity. How could you increase the activity demands to enhance the challenge and further nurture Tina's motor and process performance skills?

9. Although ABC Day Care and Kindergarten has supplies for many crafts, the tissue art project (see Figures 8.4 and 8.5); the Woodsies™ character patterns, a wood craft project (Forster Inc.®; see Figure 8.6); and Puzzle Power™ (S&S; see Figure 8.7) catch

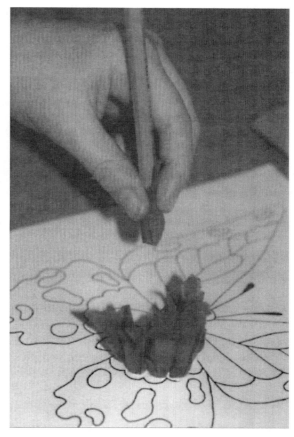

Figure 8.4. Sample tissue art project (S&S Worldwide). Reproduced with permission.

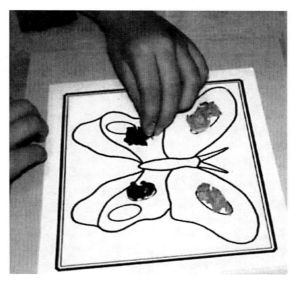

Figure 8.5. Sample tissue art project (S&S Worldwide). Reproduced with permission.

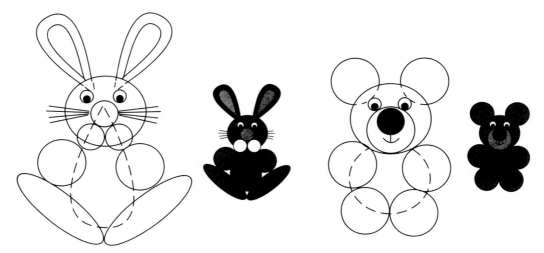

Figure 8.6. Woodsies™ Character Patterns (Forster Inc.): A wood craft project. Reproduced with permission. Forster Inc., P.O. Box 657, Wilton, ME 04294.

your attention. As with the therapeutic activity of the sunflower craft, the purpose of these projects is to enhance participation in student activities and the education occupation by promoting the development of specific client factors and performance skills. The focus of this remediation or restoration approach to therapy is to change client factors and establish a skill or ability that has not yet been developed. What features of these activities make them particularly attractive for use with children with limitations in motor and process performance skills?

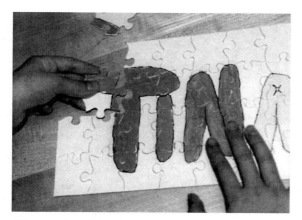

Figure 8.7. Sample Puzzle Power™ (S&S Worldwide) project. Reproduced with permission.

After analyzing these activities for their potential to address intervention objectives aimed at Tina's goals, you realize that adjustments can be made to maximize therapeutic value. Explain how the activity demands of these projects can be adjusted to ensure success while challenging Tina. Explain why purposeful activities can balance achievement with challenge. Would you recommend assistive equipment to support Tina's efforts to improve her skills, such as pencil grips or specially designed scissors? The compensatory or adaptation approach to therapy guides occupational therapy practitioners in revising the current context or activity demands to support performance in natural settings.

10. Role-play Tina and her occupational therapy practitioner with another person. This will increase the accuracy of your task and activity analysis and enable you to practice the communication and interaction style you might use with a young child. The verbal and nonverbal interactive relationship between therapist and client provides a source of encouragement, motivation, and feedback to reinforce and facilitate learning.

11. Assume that the case manager has asked for consultation regarding how ABC Day Care

and Kindergarten might provide an enriched environment and therapeutic activity experiences to enhance the performance of all children while integrating strategies for children with special needs. What therapeutic activities would you recommend that the staff at ABC Day Care and Kindergarten integrate into their activity planning? What recommendations do you have regarding enrichments to the social and cultural context to promote the healthy development of all children to enhance their occupational performance at school?

12. Explore the process of integrating the person–environment–occupation model of practice with the frame of reference outlined in the *Occupational Therapy Practice Framework,* which further guides evaluation and intervention. Models of practice give general guidance for practice, explain complex relations among concepts, and are "a set of ideas derived from various fields of study which are organized to form a synthesis and integration of elements of theory and practice" (Hagedorn, 1997, p. 144). By comparison, frames of reference reflect the knowledge and theories within the basic sciences and provide a paradigm through which practitioners view the world, solve problems, and prescribe solutions (Hagedorn, 1997). Research and indentify frames of reference used in occupational therapy. What frames of reference could you use to interpret Tina's occupational performance profile in the education occupation?

13. According to the U.S. Department of Education, 12.2 percent of students enrolled in American schools in 1993–94 were officially designated as having disabilities, and 5.3 million children and adolescents participated in federally funded programs for students with disabilities (Kaye, 1997). As an occupational therapy practitioner, how might you contribute to the promotion of health among this population?

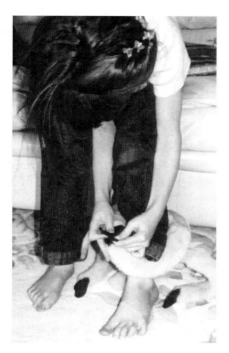

 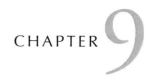

Activities of Daily Living as Occupation

Occupational therapists feel that everyday activities are significant and meaningful. They have a firm belief that it is important to be able to perform everyday activities and that those activities are essential to one's sense of self-worth.

—Flemming, 1994, p. 104

CHAPTER OBJECTIVES
■ To describe how occupational therapy practitioners can use task analysis as an evaluation and intervention tool when identifying intervention strategies to enable young clients to participate in activities of daily living.
■ To define process performance skills, client factors, and contexts as dimensions of occupational therapy.
■ To apply task analysis to the challenge of profiling the performance patterns, process performance skills, and client factors that are challenged during participation in a basic activity of daily living.

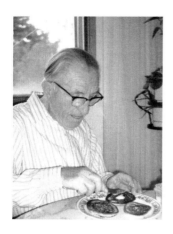

Activities of Daily Living as Occupation

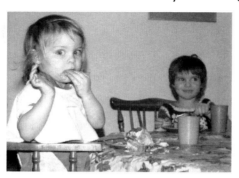

According to the Bureau of the Census (1997), 9.1 percent—almost one in 10—children younger than age 14 in the United States in 1997 had some level of disability, and 1.1 percent of children had a severe disability. Furthermore, 52.6 million people (19.7 percent of the population) older than age 15 had a disability, and 33.0 million (12.3 percent) had a severe disability. About 10.1 million people needed personal assistance with one or more activities of daily living (ADL) (McNeil, 1997). When researchers at the Census Bureau calculated these statistics, they considered a person to have a disability if he or she had difficulty performing certain sensory and motor functions, ADL, or certain social roles. A person was considered to have a severe disability if he or she was unable to perform one or more ADL, used an assistive device to get around, or needed assistance from another person to perform basic ADL (Bureau of the Census, 1997).

Clearly, the concept of disability is tied to participation in ADL. This is not surprising, given that participation in this area of occupation supports a person's integration into their social world; this integration influences self-esteem and personal identity and affords a sense of dignity, self-esteem, belonging, and meaning.

ADL is the area of occupation that supports effective living. Basic activities of daily living (BADL), sometimes called "personal activities of daily living," include self-care activities such as bathing, showering, dressing, eating, and hygiene. By comparison, instrumental activities of daily living (IADL) are the more complex activities necessary to maintain independence and live effectively in the home and community. IADL include caring for others, child rearing, pet care, meal preparation and cleanup, financial management, home establishment and maintenance, and health management (American Occupational Therapy Association [AOTA], 2002). These areas of occupation are defined in Appendix A.

To engage in daily living activities, children must acquire the requisite performance skills (i.e., process, motor, and communication and interaction skills) and performance patterns (i.e., roles, routines, and habits). Children begin to acquire these skills and patterns early in life, and they continue to refine them throughout adolescence and adulthood. Children learn through participation when parents and others guide the learning process by teaching, coaching, and cueing. In this way toddlers practice and eventually learn how to hold a cup, finger feed and use a spoon, wipe their face and hands, brush their teeth, and so forth. Over time, school-age children become more skilled in bathing and showering, managing personal hygiene, grooming, and other such activities. The development of proficiency in BADL largely occurs from 3 years to early adolescence. Adolescents continue to refine their performance skills through enhanced participation in personal care and IADL. During adulthood, skills are refined that are required for IADL such as child rearing, caring for others, and home and financial management.

BADL routines typically occur every day according to repetitive sequences. Over time children develop their performance skills and create their own routines and habits of engagement (i.e., performance patterns). The acquisition of performance skills and patterns related to BADL that began when children imitate their parents engaging in these occupations continues during playtime when children rehearse these skills by putting costumes on and taking them off, grooming dolls when playing house, and performing similar activities. The *International Classification of Functioning, Disability and Health* defined the process of copying, rehearsing, and acquiring skills as a dimension of learning and the application of knowledge (World Health Organization [WHO], 2001, p. 96). *Copying* is a basic component of learning and is defined as imitating or mimicking. Children imitate simple motor actions between ages 1 and 2 years. They can be observed copying their parents at the dinner table as they learn to use utensils and in the bathroom as they brush their teeth during morning routines. *Rehearsing* is defined as the repetition of a sequence of events, and children can be observed rehearsing BADL in their role-play and imaginary activities.

Although children acquire performance patterns and skills required for ADL as a natural part of growth and development, the complexity of the interactive learning process is often taken for granted. Occupational therapy practitioners are aware of this complexity when they observe clients as they engage in ADL, and practitioners use task analysis during evaluation to untangle this complex interaction among performance skills and patterns, contextual dimensions, activity demands, and client factors. In addition, practitioners use ADL as an occupation-based activity or purposeful activity during the intervention phase of therapy to promote engagement and participation. Activity demands and contexts are critical considerations during evaluation and intervention. For example, activity demands such as required tools and materials, environmental contexts such as social supports, and personal contexts such as expectations will support or hinder participation. In essence, people acquire performance skills through participation in ADL, and because engagement promotes development, it can be used as a health intervention.

This chapter provides readers an opportunity in the case study of Miguel to use task analysis to increase their understanding of a child's participation in the ADL area of occupation and the development of requisite performance skills and patterns. For Miguel to fully participate in the ADL occupation, he must develop several performance skills. Readers will establish an occupational profile and an analysis of Miguel's performance to identify the performance skills and patterns, contexts, activity demands, and client factors that affect his participation in ADL. A priority for the family is Miguel's development of independence with feeding, dressing, and toileting.

Dimensions of Engagement and Participation

All of the dimensions of occupational performance influence a person's participation in the ADL occupation: performance skills and patterns, contexts, activity demands, and client factors. This chapter focuses on process performance skills, client factors (sensory and motor functions), and contexts that influence Miguel's participation in ADL.

Performance Skills

As described more fully in chapter 7 and Appendix B, motor performance skills are what one does, and

CASE STUDY: MIGUEL

Miguel is a 5-year-old boy who was referred for occupational therapy services by his preschool teacher. Sue is an occupational therapy practitioner who provides evaluation and intervention services to ABC Preschool and Day Care. Miguel's teacher observed his preschool performance throughout the fall and expressed concern about general delays in Miguel's participation in ADL; development of fine-motor and gross-motor skills; and acquisition of preschool concepts such as colors, numbers, and shapes. Sue requested that the teacher and Miguel's parents get together to gather and share information regarding Miguel's occupational history and levels of participation in preschool activities. Miguel's grand-

parents expressed an interest in attending the meeting.

At the meeting, Sue learned about Miguel's developmental history. He sat at 12 months, crawled at 14 months, and walked at 20 months. He was a happy toddler who was content to listen to music and play with his toys. He was difficult to toilet train and eventually accomplished the skill at age 4.

Miguel's family had established daily routines and habits for his care. Both parents leave home for work at 6:00 a.m. before Miguel wakes. His grandparents live with the family and care for Miguel in the morning. Grandfather wakes him and ensures that Miguel eats his breakfast. Miguel has difficulty using a spoon and often resorts to finger feeding. Miguel has a

tendency to be distracted from this and other tasks, and each morning it is reinforced that he can watch a bit of TV if he finishes breakfast, grooms, and dresses for school. His grandmother dresses and grooms Miguel because he needs maximum assistance with initiating or completing the steps of putting clothes on and brushing his teeth. Both grandparents expressed concern that Miguel's ADL skills are delayed compared to the six children they raised.

Miguel attends ABC Preschool from 9:00 a.m. until 3:00 p.m., when his mother picks him up. His father returns from work in time to join the family for dinner. His parents report that Miguel has shown little developmental progress in ADL since he was 3½ years old. Miguel's teacher

they relate to observable elements of action such as posture, mobility, coordination, strength and effort, and energy (AOTA, 2002). Motor performance skills are integral to the performance of BADL. For example, dressing requires a high level of mobility, coordination, strength, and energy, and undressing requires one to change position from standing to sitting and vice versa; get items to and from dresser drawers; and move, transport, lift, and grasp objects. Putting on trousers, socks, or shoes requires a person to stabilize, shift weight, reach, and bend. Fastening buttons and zippers requires bilateral coordination and the ability to grasp small objects.

People typically develop a dressing routine that they follow each time they dress, and they structure their environment to support this performance pattern. Changes in contextual or client factors may alter a person's ability to participate in BADL (and other areas of occupations), and he or she will have to adapt to new routines.

Process performance skills are used in managing and modifying actions to participate in tasks. These skills include the following:

- Energy, required to sustain effort over the course of the activity (i.e., paces and attends)
- Knowledge acquisition (i.e., chooses, uses, handles, heeds, and inquires)
- Temporal organization pertaining to the beginning, logical order, continuation, and completion of the steps in the action sequence (i.e., initiates, continues, sequences, and terminates)
- Organization of space and objects (i.e., searches or locates, gathers, organizes, restores, and navigates)
- Adaptation by anticipating, correcting for, and benefiting by learning from consequences of errors (i.e., notices or responds, accommodates, adjusts, and benefits) (AOTA, 2002).

Like motor performance skills, process performance skills are integral to participation in ADL. To care for teeth and skin, for example, one reported that he has difficulty with putting his coat and shoes on, putting his shoes on the right feet, using the hook-and-loop fastenings on his shoes, and managing his clothing during toileting.

Miguel's preschool teacher shared with the parents her observations that he is continually engaged in classroom activities and interested in playing with his peers. She reported that he loves books about animals and "building houses like my Dad" with large foam blocks. She shared her concerns about his balance and coordination in gross-motor activities, fine-motor skill development, and knowledge of basic academic concepts.

Sue observed Miguel in the preschool and noted that he could not orient his coat and shoes to put them on correctly and did not attempt to do the zipper. His body posture and movement suggested that he had low body tone that affected his ability to balance. For example, when he threw a ball and shifted his weight forward, he fell. Miguel held a crayon with an immature palmar grasp, and his pictures looked like random squiggles. When asked to draw a picture of a boy, Miguel's illustration consisted of a circle for a head, random smaller circles for facial features, and lines extending out from the head for limbs. Miguel tried to cut out his drawing of a boy with scissors, but he could not cut along a thick line when Sue drew a frame around his picture. Miguel recognized his favorite color, green, but was inconsistent when Sue asked him to identify the colors of his crayons. When Sue asked him to count his crayons, Miguel missed numbers in an attempt to count 10 of them. When she drew pictures, Miguel correctly identified a circle and square but could not label the triangle or rectangle. He quickly became bored with the activity.

Sue completed a formal evaluation with Miguel outside of the classroom to reduce environmental distractions. The formal evaluation identified fine- and gross-motor foundation abilities at a 3½-year level, low body tone, decreased balance and equilibrium, poor manual dexterity, and delays in visual perceptual (developmental age of 3.2 years) and visual motor (developmental age of 4.1) development, with the greatest weakness in spatial relations and sequencing. ■

---

must know what to do, initiate the action of doing, sequence the steps such as retrieving the toothpaste and soap, and organize the required space and objects. People learn and rehearse these process skills as children. The more complex process skills of IADL such as child rearing, community mobility, and home management must be learned and rehearsed as adolescents and adults. Process performance skills are defined in Appendix B.

Client Factors

Client factors are "those factors that reside within the client and that may affect performance in areas of occupation" and include body functions and structures (AOTA, 2002 p. 613). Body functions are the physiological functions of body systems and include psychological functions. Body structures are "anatomical parts of the body such as organs, limbs and their components that support body function" (WHO, 2001, p. 10).

Occupational therapy practitioners evaluate body functions and structures because people need these client factors to engage in occupations. Practitioners' knowledge of these client factors enables them to identify the body functions and structures that might change as a result of participation in therapeutic activities. There is clearly an interaction between performance skills and client factors. Client factors are defined in Appendix F.

Contexts

The importance clients place on participation in ADL and self-care activities is influenced by environmental and personal contexts. Activities are culturally prescribed, and what defines an activity is laden with cultural values about the "right" way to do something. These cultural definitions and values can act as "time-tested guides to occupational experience or as oppressive systems that limit freedom and creativity" (Pierce, 2001,

p. 138). Cultural role expectations govern the norms of participation, and persons outside the norm, as are those who have diminished self-care abilities, may be stigmatized (Christiansen & Baum, 1997; Mosey, 1996). Social stigma significantly influences identity; "identity can be viewed as the super ordinate view of ourselves that includes both self-esteem and self-concept, but also importantly reflects and is influenced by the larger social world in which we find ourselves" (Christiansen, 1999, p. 549).

Personal and environmental contextual dimensions involve a variety of interrelated conditions within and surrounding the client that influence his or her performance. These contexts affect the development and acquisition of performance skills and patterns and may influence activity demands (e.g., social demands). The cultural, physical, and social contexts form the background for ADL as they dictate customs, norms, beliefs, role expectations, and social routines, as well as define the terrain and structure of the environment. A thorough list of performance context definitions is provided in Appendix D.

The Challenge

1. What is the developmental sequence and timing for the acquisition of different BADL?
2. How do the social norms for ADL vary across subcultures within the United States? How do these norms vary among countries such as the United States, Australia, Canada, England, France, Germany, or any other country with which you are familiar?
3. Review and refamiliarize yourself with Figure 3.2 and the definition of terms from *Occupational Therapy Practice Framework: Domain and Process* (AOTA, 2002; see Appendixes B–F).
4. Read the case study of Miguel and complete the Client Profile and Task Analysis Form provided in Appendix J. Complete the Activity Demand section of the form by analyzing the task of putting underwear, pants, and a T-shirt on and taking them off.

5. Table 9.1 suggests some client goals for Miguel. Define one or more additional goals and objectives. A suggested format for writing client goals is provided in Appendix K. In practice, you would establish these goals and objectives in collaboration with Miguel's family, teacher, and any other caregivers.
6. Design an occupation-based therapeutic activity for Miguel to do during one 30-minute session to address one of the goals. This purposeful activity should (a) address the concerns and priorities of this family and teacher; (b) meet the developmental needs of this child; and (c) satisfy the criteria for a purposeful activity as delineated by AOTA (1993). What approaches to occupational therapy intervention have you used to address this goal (see Appendix G)?
7. Design an occupation-based activity for Miguel to do at home with his family. What approaches to occupational therapy intervention have you used (see Appendix G)?
8. Explore the process of integrating the person–environment–occupation model of practice with the frame of reference outlined in the *Occupational Therapy Practice Framework,* which further guides evaluation and intervention. Models of practice give general guidance for practice, explain complex relations among concepts, and are "a set of ideas derived from various fields of study which are organized to form a synthesis and integration of elements of theory and practice" (Hagedorn, 1997, p. 144). By comparison, frames of reference reflect the knowledge and theories within the basic sciences and provide a paradigm through which practitioners view the world, solve problems, and prescribe solutions (Hagedorn, 1997). Research and identify frames of reference used in occupational therapy. What frames of reference could you use to interpret Miguel's occupational performance profile in the occupation of ADL?
9. There are many children, adolescents, and adults who have limitations in ADL. How

Table 9.1. Client goals for Miguel.

Long-Term Goal	Short-Term Objectives
1. Miguel will independently put his clothes on during his morning routine by the beginning of kindergarten (in 8 months).	1a. Miguel will improve his ability to put on his underwear and T-shirt from maximum to minimum assistance with cueing (within 6 months).
	1b. Miguel will improve his ability to put his coat on from maximum to minimum assistance with cueing (within 6 months).
	1c.
2. Miguel will improve his fine-motor dexterity through practice while learning how to fasten large buttons and hook-and-loop fastenings on his shoes, and these improved skills will transfer to his ability to manipulate crayons and scissors.	2a. Miguel will learn to unfasten large buttons on a play button board within 2 months and will transfer the skills to unfastening his pajama tops within 6 months.
	2b. Miguel will pull up the zipper on his jacket once it is started (within 1 month).
3.	3a.
	3b.
4.	4a.
	4b.

might a school (e.g., parent–teacher association) or community (e.g., boys and girls club) group support the ADL occupation among the population? Consider how these organizations could influence activity demands and environmental contexts in support of a goal to enhance engagement of children in ADL and IADL occupations. How might these groups collaborate to define goals, objectives, and an implementation plan to contribute to a reduction in limitations and participation restrictions in this area? ■

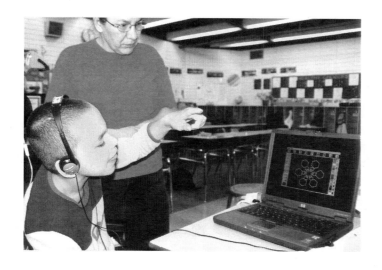

CHAPTER 10

Assistive Technology in Education

It is doubtful that any child may reasonably be expected to succeed in life if he is denied the opportunity of an education. Such an opportunity, where the state has undertaken to provide it, is a right which must be made available to all on equal terms.

—Brown v. Board of Education, *1954*

CHAPTER OBJECTIVES

▪ To describe the relevance of assistive technology to participation in education.

▪ To describe the occupational profile of a young client and the use of task analysis in evaluation and intervention with a child who has a disability.

▪ To discuss ways to use logical thinking and creative analysis to alter activity demands and restructure environmental contexts to enhance a client's participation by means of assistive technology.

▪ To distinguish remedial and compensation approaches to intervention that address the consequences of impairment and disability.

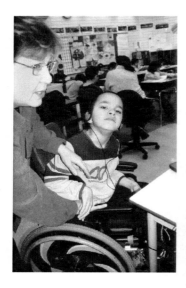

Assistive Technology in Education

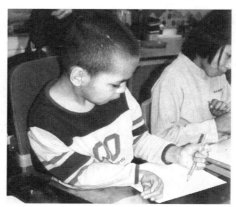

The versatile nature of technology has provided educators with greater flexibility in customizing and individualizing educational strategies for all students and in restructuring the contexts of learning and classrooms. The availability and accessibility of technological devices enables teachers to formulate learning goals that maximize the potential for all learners, including those who have a disability (Center for Applied Technology [CAST], 2002). Assistive technology can be considered a scaffold on which students with (or without) disabilities can participate in education. The opportunity to engage in tasks using assistive technology is motivating to students and provides opportunities to practice, receive immediate feedback, and demonstrate skills. Occupational therapy practitioners help clients use assistive technology to engage in occupations (American Occupational Therapy Association [AOTA], 2002).

Assistive technology refers to a broad range of devices, services, strategies, and practices that are conceived and applied to ameliorate the problems faced by individuals who have disabilities. An assistive technology *device* is "any item, piece of equipment, or product system, whether acquired commercially, modified, or customized, that is used to increase, maintain, or improve functional capacities of individuals with disabilities," and an assistive technology *service* "directly assists an individual with a disability in the selection, acquisition, or use of an assistive technology device" (Individuals With Disabilities Education Act [IDEA], 1990; Assistive Technology Act, 1998). Assistive technology devices are an integral part of special education and the individualized education program (IDEA, 1990).

Assistive technology has evolved over time to include both low-technology and high-technology devices. Low-technology devices are simple to program and inexpensive and include such things as typing and writing aids. High-technology devices are more expensive, complicated, and customizable, and many include such features as switches, computers, power wheelchairs, and environmental control units (ECUs). Children and adults who have a constellation of activity limitations can maximize their participation in day-to-day occupations with the use of assistive technology. For example, ECUs can enable children to manage their environments by remote control and to maintain an interest in interacting with their world. There is some evidence that the use of assistive technology may prevent learned helplessness in some children (Swinth, 1996).

Public policy has created a social and political context that ensures equal access to education and learning opportunities. For example, IDEA (1990), the Rehabilitation Act (1973), the Assistive Technology Act (1998), and the Americans With Disabilities Act (1990) have provided the legislative and regulatory frameworks for the expression of this public value. IDEA ensures that students with disabilities have access to free appropriate public education and requires school districts to provide assistive technology devices and services to individual students if the team determines the child has a need. The Rehabilitation Act states that no person with a disability shall be excluded from participation, denied benefits, or otherwise subjected to discrimination because of his or her disability. The Assistive Technology Act assists each state in maintaining and strengthening a permanent comprehensive statewide program of technology-related assistance for persons of all ages who have a disability. The Americans with Disabilities Act states that local counties or state governments must make facilities and services accessible to persons with disabilities.

Assistive Technology in Education

Assistive technology, even high-technology devices such as computers, cannot substitute for intervention directed toward changing curricular demands through the creation of individual education plans and altering classroom environments to be more enabling for all students (CAST, 2002). Indeed, changes to activity demands and environments may result in more appropriate contexts and less requirements for assistive technology. Whereas the use of assistive technology focuses responsibility for adaptation on the child, the alteration of activity demands and environmental contexts focuses responsibility for adaptation on others. The key to services for children who have disabilities is to apply the principles of participation and engagement; best fit of strate-

gies, techniques, and devices; and diversity in approaches.

Health practitioners must be careful when recommending the use of assistive technology devices to ensure that they are not seen as substitutes for other initiatives that foster greater engagement of students in the curriculum and classroom. For example, it is easy to assume that the use of a software program will enable a student with disabilities to learn concepts, but children (and adults) typically need to learn, rehearse, and generalize concepts through participation in a full range of activities. Assistive technology devices prepare clients for more purposeful and occupation-based activities. Clients will not improve the performance skills and client factors they need for engagement in the full range of education occupations exclusively through the use of assistive technology; they will improve these skills and factors through engagement in curricular and classroom activities.

This chapter provides readers an opportunity to use task analysis as an evaluation and intervention tool to profile a client's participation in the education occupation using the case study of Sidney. Readers will establish an occupational profile and an analysis of Sidney's performance to identify her interests, values, and needs, as well as the performance patterns and skills, contexts, activity demands, and client factors that affect her participation. For Sidney to fully participate in the occupation of education, activity demands must be altered and environmental contexts addressed. Assistive technology devices such as switches have the potential to facilitate Sidney's engagement in meaningful occupations and to promote further development of performance patterns and skills.

Use of Assistive Technology to Enhance Participation

According to the World Health Organization (WHO, 2001), "Restrictions in participation in education are brought about by the features of the physical and social environment of a person that make it difficult, or perhaps impossible, to have the opportunity to learn and to perform in the educa-

CASE STUDY: SIDNEY

Sidney was diagnosed with spastic cerebral palsy and developmental delay at a young age. She is now 7 years old and has just moved to a new school district. She has a manual wheelchair for functional and community mobility but is unable to propel independently. Sidney's upper and lower limbs are hypertonic, but her trunk is hypotonic. She has poor postural stability and is unable to sit independently. When her head and trunk are reclined toward supine, Sidney's arms extend and her lower extremities extend, abduct, and internally rotate. Her current wheelchair has a special seating insert that positions her hips, knees, and ankles at 90 degrees of flexion. The insert has lateral supports, and the seat and back cushions are firm. Her speech is unintelligible to people who are not accustomed to listening to her speak.

At age 4 years, Sidney began learning to use a switch to control her environment and participate in new activities. She has progressed from using one vertical-toggle single switch to using two single switches (2-in. diameter) that are attached to her wheelchair tray. She uses these switches to operate toys, a radio, and some kitchen appliances. Throughout the day, Sidney tends to rest her arms in a flexed position on her wheelchair tray. When she reaches for her switch, Sidney internally rotates and slightly flexes her shoulder and extends her elbow. She depresses the switch with a fisted grasp pattern. Sidney remains nonverbal but uses a basic communication board that has slots for four 3-in. pictures. Sidney has a collection of approximately 15 pictures that represent people and activities that interest her, but only four pictures can be used on her board at one time. When provided with smaller pictures, Sidney's reach is occasionally inaccurate, making it difficult to determine which pictures she is selecting.

Sidney's parents are interested in incorporating switch use into Sidney's educational curriculum and have asked for an occupational therapy practitioner to provide suggestions to the classroom teacher and others in the school. One of the goals on Sidney's individualized education program is to maximize her participation in classroom learning experiences. The teacher at ABC Elementary has limited experience with assistive technology devices and would like you to provide specific activity recommenda-

tion setting" (p. 153). The consequence of an impairment of body function or body structure may be disability; limitations and restrictions may arise as a direct consequence of impairments at the organ level or as the person's response to the impairment (WHO, 1980). Many persons have disabilities, activity limitations, and participation restrictions as a result of impairments that can be ameliorated through the application of preparatory methods or purposeful activities using a remedial or restorative approach to intervention.

For persons whose disabilities result from impairments that cannot be ameliorated through the application or use of these interventions, services are directed toward altering activity demands or environmental contexts to promote participation. For example, some children are not able to articulate speech clearly, and they can use assistive technology to communicate. Similarly, some children do not have the upper-limb control and hand dexterity to operate a standard computer keyboard, and assistive technology (e.g., switches or voice recognition software) can help them operate devices such as a computer. This approach to intervention is referred to as compensation or adaptation (Appendix G), and the expected outcome of intervention is enhanced occupational performance (i.e., the ability to carry out important activities of daily life) and role competence (i.e., the ability to effectively meet the demands of roles in which the client engages) (AOTA, 2002).

The role of the occupational therapy practitioner is to ensure that not all impairments restrict participation in meaningful occupations. The practitioner may be able to use assistive technology to alter activity demands and restructure environmental contexts. This approach to intervention enables clients to minimize the impact of the disability and promotes adaptation. Assistive tions. He also indicates a preference for switch activities that fit into regular weekly scheduled art, science, math, music, and physical education classes. Sidney is the only child with cerebral palsy in her school, and to date communication strategies have not developed to enable her to verbally interact with her peers.

Sidney's home life centers on sports and recreation. Her father is a baseball coach, and her brother plays baseball and soccer. Sidney loves to attend the games and screams for her brother from the sidelines when he scores a goal. Her mother works full-time at a local bakery and sends Sidney to school with freshly baked cookies every Monday. Sidney uses the Power-Link 3 Control Unit (AbleNet Inc.) at home with kitchen appliances to bake with her mother. Her father has at-tached a switch to a red rotating light that Sidney activates during exciting moments at baseball or soccer games.

Learning Resources

AbleNet: www.ablenetinc.com

Alliance for Technology Access: www.ataccess.org

Americans With Disabilities Act: www.ada.org

Assistive Technology Act: www.resna.org/ata

Assistive Technology Training Online Project: www.atto.buffalo.edu

Center for Special Technology: www.cast.org

Closing the Gap: Computer Technology in Special Education and Rehabilitation: www.closingthegap.com

Individuals With Disabilities Education Act: www.ideapractices.org,

www.ed.gov/offices/OSERS/Policy/IDEA/the_law.html

Network of Regional Technology in Education Consortia: www.rtec.org

President's Commission on Excellence in Special Education: www.ed.gov/inits/commissions boards/whspecialeducation

Rehabilitation Act: www.ed.gov/offices/OSERS/RSA

Rehabilitation Engineering and Rehabilitation Society of North America: www.resna.org

Tash International Inc.: www.tashinc.com

Toys for Special Children and Enabling Devices: www.enabling.com ■

technology may also be used as a purposeful activity to establish or restore performance skills, particularly in the motor and communication dimensions. In this context, assistive technology is used as a preparatory method for remediation or restoration of client skills or abilities (AOTA, 2002) (see Appendixes G and H).

Task analysis can assist practitioners in constructing an occupational profile of performance patterns and skills, environmental and personal contexts, activity demands, and client factors. This information provides a basis for intervention planning to ensure the useful and appropriate application of technology. The client and family guide the use of technology in intervention planning and implementation according to their values and needs, sociocultural and environmental factors, financial resources, and the cost-effectiveness of the technology (AOTA, 1991; Shuster, 1993; Swinth, 1996). When planning an inter-vention, practitioners should keep in mind that learning to use assistive technology will be a slow process for the learner both physically and cognitively. Therefore, the intervention plan and the recommended technology should be attractive, motivating, and engaging for the client.

Switch Access to Educational Experiences

There are several devices that children use, such as toys, computers, and television, that are operated (i.e., turned on and off) and controlled (e.g., volume, channel) by switches. To ensure that persons with physical disabilities are able to operate these devices and participate in the occupations associated with their use, there are several switches that are commercially available in different shapes, colors, and sizes for use by people with varying abilities (see Figure 10.1 and Table 10.1). The goals of the client guide decisions regarding the use of a switch or switches. The client's performance skills

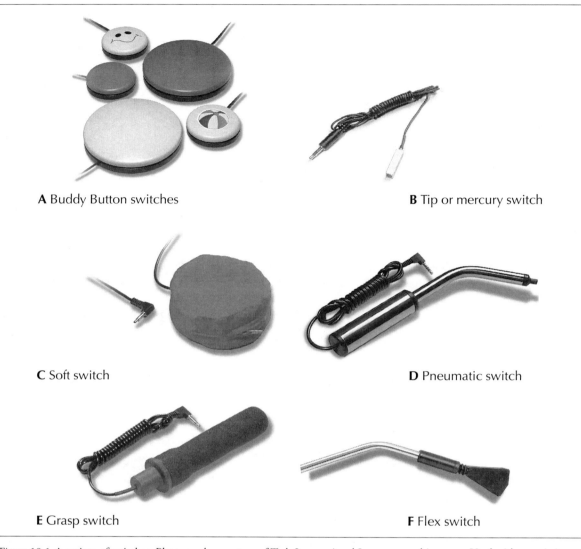

A Buddy Button switches

B Tip or mercury switch

C Soft switch

D Pneumatic switch

E Grasp switch

F Flex switch

Figure 10.1. A variety of switches. Photographs courtesy of Tash International Inc., www.tashinc.com. Used with permission.

and contexts influence decisions about the desired features of assistive technology devices.

Switches function as on–off devices to enable clients of all ages to activate battery-operated and electrical appliances such as toys, fans, and door openers. Switches can also be used for more complex devices such as radios, computers, televisions, power wheelchairs, and home appliances. Children as young as ages 6–9 months can control switch access to toys and computer cause-and-effect programs (Glickman, Deitz, Anson, & Stewart, 1996; Swinth, Anson, & Deitz, 1993).

Switches connected to ECUs allow individuals with disabilities to maintain a more independent level of activity and engagement.

All battery-operated toys and appliances require activation of an on–off switch that closes an electrical circuit to supply a motor with power. Typical on–off switches require fine-motor coordination and strength. By changing the on–off control to an alternative switch, the size and location of the activation device can be altered; this modification thus alters the demands of the activity. Several manufacturers make toys and other battery-

Table 10.1. Commonly used switches and interfaces.

Name/Example	Activation	Comments	Vendors
Flat Switch	Small low-force movement of arms, hands, legs, head, etc.	• flatness allows placement under many objects • notebook switch provides larger surfaces	Don Johnson Tash
Leaf Switch	Flexible switch that is activated when bent or pressed gently.	• requires mounting • can improve head control and fine motor skills	Don Johnson Tash Enabling Devices
Mecury (Tilt) Switch	Gravity-sensitive switch activates when tilted beyond a certain point.	• can improve head or other posture control • attaches easily with Velcro® strap	HCTS Tash Enabling Devices
Plate Switch—Rectangular	Downward pressure on plate by hand, foot, arm, leg, or other reliable movement.	• most common • can be covered with various textures • some offer light, music, vibration, vertical position	Don Johnson Tash Enabling Devices
Plate Switch—Circular	Light touch anywhere on the top of surface.	• recommended for young children • click provides auditory feedback • 5" diameter and smaller size available	Ablenet Tash
Voice Activated	Significant vocalizations (1–2 seconds) required.	• can improve vocalizations sound sensitivity control	Enabling Devices
Wobble Switch	Requires slight press to midline for activation; audible click.	• versatile and multi-faceted • available with goose-neck positioner • sturdy	Prentke-romich Enabling Devices
Puzzle switch	Pieces must be properly inserted to activate toy.	• ideal for introducing children to basic cognitive concepts • can improve fine motor skills • complexity of task can be varied	Enabling Devices

Continued

Note. From "Using Assistive Technology for Play and Learning: Children, From Birth to 10 Years of Age" (pp. 131–163), by S. G. Mistrett and S. J. Lane, 1995, in *Assistive Technology for Persons with Disability* (4th ed.), edited by W. Mann and J. Lane, Bethesda, MD: American Occupational Therapy Association. Copyright 1995 by the American Occupational Therapy Association. Reproduced with permission.

Table 10.1. Commonly used switches and interfaces *(continued)*.

Name/Example	Activation	Comments	Vendors
Battery Device Adapter	Allows a battery-operated device to be activated by a switch.	• nonpermanent • can be used with most on–off toys, radios, and tape recorders	AbleNet Don Johnson Enabling Devices
Computer Switch Interface	Allows a single-switch access to an Apple computer.	• accepts one or two switches • substitute switches for joy-sticks	AbleNet Don Johnson Tash
Control Unit	Enables electrical devices to be activated by a switch.	• allows children to participate with peers • used with continuous closure or on–off • timer can be set from 2–90 seconds	AbleNet Don Johnson Tash
Series Adapter	Connects two switches and one toy. Both switches must be activated at the same time.	• encourages bilateral movement • promotes cooperation between two children	Don Johnson HCTS Enabling Devices
Switch Latch Interface	Turns the device on and off with each switch activation.	• good for children who are unable to maintain switch closure for any length of time	AbleNet Don Johnson HCTS Enabling Devices
Timer Module	When switch is closed, a toy is activated for a preset time.	• the toy activates for 1–90 seconds, depending on the vendor	AbleNet HCTS Enabling Devices
Jack Adapter	Works to convert the size of the jack to the size required by the toy or device.	• must be mono to work with switches	Radio Shack

operated appliances with external switch jacks. Other devices have switches permanently attached. Some switches provide sensory feedback by vibrating, illuminating, and playing music or making another sound. The BIGmack™ (AbleNet Inc.) single switch, for example, has 20 seconds of memory to record and play back audio messages.

A battery device adapter is a very inexpensive activation device for a battery-operated appliance with a switch. Battery device adapters have a copper wafer at one end and a plug at the other, as illustrated in Table 10.1. The copper wafer is placed between the battery and the lead on the appliance, and the on–off switch is turned on (Figure 10.2). The appliance motor will not operate because the battery device adapter has interrupted the electrical circuit. Once the switch is plugged into the battery device adapter plug and pressed, the electrical circuit is complete and the motor will operate. On–off control has been transferred from the appliance to the switch.

Switches activate battery-operated appliances only when they are depressed, unless a latch

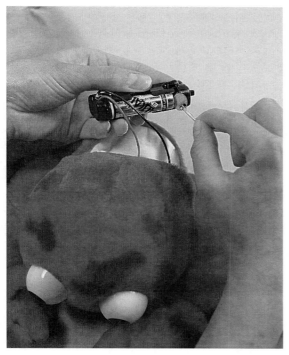

Figure 10.2. Using a battery adapter. Photograph courtesy of Tash International Inc., www.tashinc.com.

switch or a latch interface device is used. Activation of the latch switch will turn the appliance on, but a second activation will be required to turn the appliance off. A television remote control, for example, is a latch switch. An illustration of a switch latch interface is found in Table 10.1. Single, dual, and multiple switches allow clients to activate an assortment of appliances and devices. Switch software programs enable a person to press only one switch to operate the computer. The switch can be located on any one of several input devices, including the button of a joystick, a mouse, or the keyboard space bar. Children with limited motor skills can use one big button switch as the input device.

The ULTRA 4 Remote System (Tash International Inc.) is an ECU that allows remote control of electrical appliances. The ULTRA 4 contains a transmitter box with four latch switches. Four receiver boxes are plugged into the electrical receptors on the wall between the electrical appliance and the outlet. The appliance is turned on, but the motor will not operate until a switch on the transmitter box is pressed. The ULTRA 4 Remote System transfers the appliance's on–off lever to the latch switch on the transmitter. Communication between the transmitter and receivers occurs through ultrasound signals. Four different color transmitter switches operate four color-coded receivers. Figure 10.3 shows two different transmitters, and Figure 10.4 shows the Scanning ULTRA 4, a transmitter that enables a person to use four single switches or one switch to scan and select signals.

The PowerLink 3® Control Unit (AbleNet Inc.) enables direct, latch, and timed switch control of any electrical appliance. The PowerLink 3 Control Unit is plugged into the wall, and an appliance is plugged into the unit. Although the appliance on–off switch must be in the on position, the appliance motor will not operate until the switch is plugged into the unit and pressed. Direct, latch, or timed mode is selected with a dial control, but this control requires fine-motor coordination and strength. The Electra Link (Tash International Inc.)

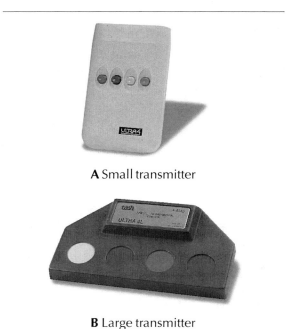

A Small transmitter

B Large transmitter

Figure 10.3. Two different transmitters for the ULTRA 4 Remote System. Photographs courtesy of Tash International Inc., www.tashinc.com.

also provides direct, latch, and timed control, but it is a wireless system that relies on infrared technology. Indeed, several ECUs use infrared to enable people to control electrical appliances (e.g., TV, DVD, lights, blinds, doors). And some units use speech recognition technology to enable persons with disabilities to control their environment.

The Challenge

1. Read the case study of Sidney and complete the Client Profile and Task Analysis Form (provided in Appendix J). Complete the occupational profile of Sidney's occupational history, interests, values, needs, and performance patterns, as well as her abilities and limitations using impairment qualifiers. Identify the activity demands and contextual variables of the classroom environment that currently challenge Sidney beyond her capabilities, and profile these factors in the sections on activity demands and required body structures and functions.

   To complete your analysis of Sidney's motor performance skills and sensory func-

tions, answer the following questions:
   a. What are your initial impressions regarding Sidney's motor performance skills and neuromusculoskeletal and movement-related body functions? Why do you think Sidney uses a wheelchair? Why does she have a special seating insert? Sidney's seating insert has a firm back and base; offers lateral support; and positions her hips, knees, and ankles in 90 degrees of flexion. Why was the insert designed with these features?
   b. What are your initial impressions regarding Sidney's process performance skills and global mental functions? Is there evidence that Sidney understands cause and effect? Do you believe that cause and effect is a prerequisite skill for the use of switches, or is it a cognitive skill that can be taught through the use of a switch? What is the advantage of using a vibrating switch to teach cause and effect?
   c. Record your impressions of the personal and environmental factors that influence Sidney's participation in meaningful occupations and of her family's insights regarding her interests, values, and needs.
2. What are the goals and priorities of this family and Sidney's teacher? Use this information to identify the performance skills and patterns, contexts, and client factors you will target during intervention. List goals and objectives for

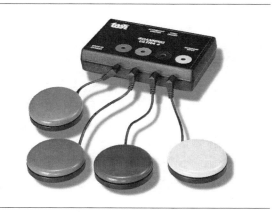

Figure 10.4. Scanning ULTRA 4 transmitter with four Buddy Button switches. Photograph courtesy of Tash International Inc., www.tashinc.com.

Table 10.2. Battery-operated or electrical appliances integrated in classroom educational activities.

Regularly Scheduled Classroom Activities	Battery-Operated or Electrical Appliances That Can Help Sidney Participate in the Activities	
	Lite Brite™	Tape Recorder
Art		
Science		
Mathematics: Learning addition and subtraction	Classmates place pegs in groups while Sidney illuminates	
Music		
Physical education		

Sidney (a sample format is provided in Appendix K). In practice, you would establish these client-centered goals in collaboration with Sidney's family and teacher, who would be her proxies.

3. Sidney's parents would like switch use to be incorporated into her educational activities. Identifying appropriate opportunities for switch use and consulting with the teacher will help you accomplish this goal. Use Table 10.2 to list all of the battery-operated and electrical appliances available in Sidney's school and educational activities and tasks that occur in typical second-grade art, science, mathematics, music, and physical education classes. How could you incorporate the use of Sidney's switch using appliances within these classes? What low-technology assistive devices are available to augment her ability to communicate with her peers?

To provide an example, if the students are painting pictures in art, Sidney could use Twirl-O-Paint® (The Ohio Art Company) for her project. During mathematics, when students are learning addition or multiplication, Sidney's classmates could place plastic pegs into grouped number clusters on a Lite Brite™ (Milton Bradley) board while Sidney activates the light mechanism to begin to learn number concepts. Read Canfield and Locke (1996) to supplement your curriculum-based classroom activity ideas.

4. Sidney uses up to two single switches and has the potential to learn how to use a voice output communication aid. This aid would enable her to scan multiple vocabulary items, which is a more complicated but efficient method of expressing information. It appears that Sidney's limited physical skills mean that she will use scanning as an access method to assistive technology in the future. It is important to note that Sidney has the potential to use more than two switches in the near future. This will require expert assessment and training. What activity would you consider having Sidney engage in to evaluate or enhance her ability to scan and use more than two switches?

5. The Rehabilitation Engineering and Rehabilitation Society of North America (RESNA) is an "interdisciplinary association of people with a common interest in technology and disability." Their "purpose is to improve the potential of people with disabilities to achieve their goals through the use of technology. [RESNA] serve[s] that purpose by promoting research, development, education, advocacy, and the provision of technology and by supporting the people engaged in these activities." RESNA posts frequently asked questions on its Web site

about access to educational technologies for students with disabilities. Reflect on the following questions as you think about the impact of technology on the performance of populations of students:

a. How do access barriers to educational technology among students with disabilities differ from barriers to access for other children?

b. How might built-in features or add-on products for computer access help all students, not just those with disabilities? *Built-in features* are components made routinely available by the manufacturer, and *add-on products* are customized components that must be purchased after (or at an extra expense at the time of) the original sale of the computer.

c. What are school's legal responsibilities to provide access to educational technologies for students with disabilities?

6. Consider the role of occupational therapy practitioners in contributing to the creation and implementation of universal design principles to enhance the engagement of persons with disabilities in their valued occupations and to contribute to the health of this population. Title II of the Assistive Technology Act of 1998 [Section 2(a)(10)] contains provisions in support of universal design:

The use of universal design principles reduces the need for many specific kinds of assistive technology devices and assistive technology services by building in accommodations for individuals with disabilities before rather than after production. The use of universal design principles also increases the likelihood that products (including services) will be compatible with existing assistive technologies. These principles are increasingly important to enhance access to information technology, telecommunications, transportation, physical structures and consumer products.... Incorporating universal design principles into the design and manufacturing of technology products, including devices of daily living ... could expand their immediate use by individuals with disabilities. [Assistive Technology Act of 1998, Section 2(a)(10)] ∎

CHAPTER 11

Computer-Assisted Engagement in Occupations

The development of machines has made muscle power obsolete and having an able body unnecessary. With modern technology, it ought to be possible for many people with disabilities to lead a life in the community and contribute to society.

—Hawking, 1996, p. 28

CHAPTER OBJECTIVES

■ To describe how a variety of computer input devices can be used to enhance participation in occupations.

■ To describe the use of task analysis in evaluation and intervention to enable a young client who has a disability to participate in meaningful occupations by means of assistive technology.

■ To discuss ways to use logical thinking and creative analysis to alter activity demands and restructure environmental contexts.

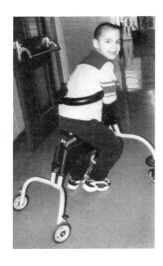

Computer-Assisted Engagement in Occupations

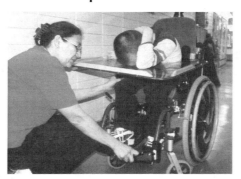

For persons who have impairments that cannot be restored through remedial or restorative approaches to intervention, assistive technology devices are an adjunctive modality that can enable them to overcome activity limitations and participation restrictions. The most commonly used devices are power wheelchairs and computers (Hawking, 1996). Power mobility is vital when the client's ambulation is limited and either upper-limb function impairment prevents the use of a manual wheelchair or lack of endurance limits community mobility. The use of assistive technology devices is an example of a preparatory method of intervention; this type of occupational therapy intervention prepares clients for more purposeful and occupation-based activities (American Occupational Therapy Association [AOTA], 2002) (see Appendix H).

Technological innovation and increased access to technology over the past two decades have provided tremendous new opportunities for persons with disabilities. According to the Assistive Technology Act of 1998,

> Technology has come to play an increasingly important role in the lives of all persons in the United States, in the conduct of business, in the functioning of government, in the fostering of communication, in the conduct

of commerce, and in the provision of education. . . . Substantial progress has been made in the development of assistive technology devices, including adaptations to existing devices that facilitate activities of daily living, that significantly benefit individuals with disabilities of all ages. Such devices and adaptations increase involvement of such individuals in, and reduce expenditures associated with, programs and activities such as early intervention, education, rehabilitation and training, employment, residential living, independent living, and recreation programs and activities, and other aspects of daily living.

Computers can be considered assistive technology devices when they are used to compensate for activity limitations and participation restrictions. Computers can be used to enhance engagement in instrumental activities of daily living, education, work, leisure, and social participation. Kaye (2000) noted that

> Computer technology and the Internet have a tremendous potential to broaden the lives and increase the independence of people with disabilities. Those who have difficulty leaving their homes can now log in and order groceries, shop for appliances, research health questions, participate in online discussions, catch up with friends, or make new ones. (p. 1)

Unfortunately, only 24 percent of persons with disabilities have a computer at home, compared to 52 percent of nondisabled people, and 11 percent have access to the Internet at home, compared to 30 percent of nondisabled people. New technologies hold great promise to enhance the population's participation in occupations, but the "computer revolution has left the vast majority of people with disabilities behind" (Kaye, 2000, p. 1). Although many persons with disabilities can use computers without altering the activity demands, some need assistive technology devices to enable access and use.

This chapter provides readers an opportunity to use task analysis in evaluation and intervention to enhance a client's participation in chosen occupations using the case study of Wayne. Wayne is having more and more difficulty engaging in an array of activities using his computer. Readers will establish an occupational profile and an analysis of Wayne's performance to identify his interests, values, and needs as well as the performance skills and patterns, contexts, and client factors that affect his participation. For Wayne to fully participate in his chosen occupations, activity demands must be altered and environmental contexts addressed to minimize participation restrictions, promote independence, enhance role performance, and maintain self-esteem.

Computers as Assistive Technology Devices

When impairments affect a person's ability to operate a conventional keyboard or mouse, an alternative computer input device is required. *Peripheral devices,* or "peripherals," are equipment that is used to interact with the computer. The keyboard and mouse are the most commonly available peripheral input devices, and other devices are available to assist clients with disabili-ties in using computers and conventional keyboards. Head sticks, mouth sticks, key guards, and typing aid orthotics are examples of low-technology devices; high-technology devices, which are more expensive and complicated, include switches, special keyboards, and special software that can be customized to meet specific needs.

There are commercially available keyboards that offer an alternative to conventional shape, size, and key locations. Miniature and expanded keyboards offer smaller- or larger-than-normal letter, numeric, and function keys. The standard key arrangement is called QWERTY, after the first five letters on the second row of the traditional keyboard (Figure 11.1). Some alternative keyboards offer a frequency-of-use layout to enhance the efficiency of movement (Figure 11.2). Alternative input computer devices include ultrasonic and infrared head pointers, voice controls, and switches. Indirect-control switch interface systems, such as the Discover:Kenx system, allow users to operate a computer using switches (Figure 11.3). These systems also allow users to create and print custom overlays for programmable keyboards; use on-screen keyboard displays, scanning, and Morse code to operate software programs; and produce speech output.

Use of Task Analysis to Enhance Participation Using Assistive Technology

When the use of assistive technology is being considered for a person with disabilities, an interdisciplinary team of professionals conducts a comprehensive evaluation and establishes and implements intervention plans that aim to establish the best fit among the person, the external environment, and the technology (Cook & Hussey, 1995; Smith, 1991). Occupational therapy practitioners often contribute their task analysis skills to interdisciplinary teams providing assistive technology services (Christiansen & Baum, 1997).

Task analysis for assistive technology use involves

- identifying activities that occur in the client's natural environment,
- determining participation restrictions and the causes of activity limitations, and
- evaluating assistive devices for their potential to promote the fit between the client and

CASE STUDY: WAYNE

Wayne is an 11-year-old boy who was diagnosed with Duchenne muscular dystrophy as a preschooler. He drives his power wheelchair to school every day using a joystick that is positioned just in front of his trunk in midline. He uses his right and left hand together to operate the joystick. Wayne has a special seating system that tilts in space. When engaging in certain activities such as computer work, Wayne prefers to have his trunk in an upright position with his hips at 90 degrees of flexion. This position is more functional for Wayne than a reclined sitting position.

Wayne has his own computer at home and school, but he is having more difficulty reaching all of the keys on both keyboards. He spends many hours throughout the week on his computer typing his schoolwork, playing computer games, surfing the Internet, and chatting with friends on e-mail. His wheelchair and computers were provided to him by community coalitions who have tried to meet his needs for assistive technology for many years. Without this assistance, Wayne's parents would not have been able to afford these expensive items.

During a recent visit to his school by an occupational therapy practitioner, Wayne indicated that the function keys at the top of the keyboard were "impossible to reach" and that the numeric keys to the far right of his keyboard were "useless." Wayne uses his left hand to push his right arm toward the function or numeric keys or leans his entire trunk to the right in an effort to reach the numeric keys. Both tasks require great effort, and when Wayne leans any distance, he is unable to return to an upright trunk position independently. When working on a lengthy project, Wayne eventually becomes very frustrated with the amount of assistance required.

Evaluation of his bilateral muscle strength indicates that Wayne has "poor minus" shoulder flexion, abduction, and external rotation. His wrist strength is poor, and his head strength is poor minus. Muscle strength qualifiers are 0 (also referred to as 0/5), poor (2/5), fair (3/5), good (4/5), and normal (5/5). The grade of 0, or poor, indicates that full range of motion occurs in a gravity-eliminated position only, and poor minus is obtained when only partial range of motion occurs in a gravity-eliminated position (Hislop & Montgomery, 1995). ∎

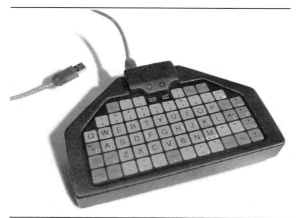

Figure 11.1. USB Mini with QWERTY layout. Photograph courtesy of Tash International Inc., www.tashinc.com.

the desired activities within customary environments.

The guiding principle is to identify accommodations that can be made without changing the critical elements of the activities; this is the basis of the match among the client, the activity, and the assistive technology device.

Practitioners evaluate clients in their customary contexts and identify performance skills and patterns, contextual resources and barriers, activity demands, and client factors that influence participation. Practitioners pay particular attention to the physical environment (e.g., classroom, workplace); currently available resources, including assistive technology and skilled personnel; and the attitudes and expectations of the client, family, and other stakeholders.

When identifying the assistive technology devices that are the most appropriate match for a client's motor and process skills and limitations, the occupational therapy practitioner considers client priorities, needs, and skills and researches the characteristics of the equipment and systems available commercially (Smith, 1991). The practitioner bases his or her recommendations on the

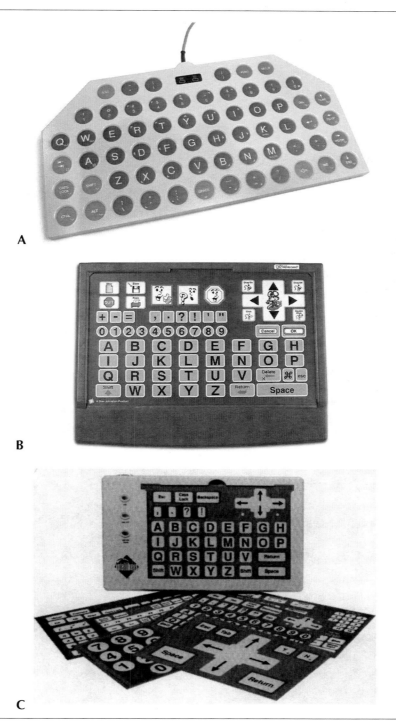

Figure 11.2. Various alternative large keyboards. (a) USB King with frequency-of-use layout. Photograph courtesy of Tash International Inc., www.tashinc.com; (b) Discover:Board. Photograph courtesy of Modentec; (c) IntelliKeys with standard overlays. Photograph courtesy of IntelliTools Inc. All rights reserved.

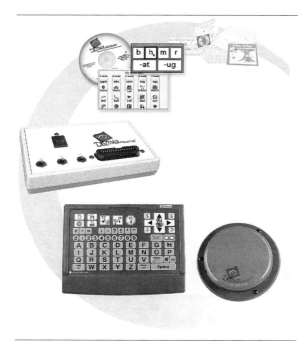

Figure 11.3. Discover:Kenx system. Photograph courtesy of Modentec.

degree of match between client and device characteristics. The practitioner may also be called on to provide training in the use of personalized systems (Dow & Rees, 1995). The client's lifestyle, interests and capabilities, roles and routines, and context are all key to the effective and appropriate use of technology.

The Importance of Partnerships

At the outset of the 21st century, it appears that technology innovations coupled with recent legislation are changing the ways that persons with disabilities engage in occupations and participate in contexts (Assistive Technology Training, 2002): "Technology has become one of the primary engines for economic activity, education, and innovation" (Assistive Technology Act, 1998). The benefits of assistive technology are most strikingly evident in the participation of persons with disabilities in the occupation of education. Public policy in support of the educational needs of children with disabilities and the use of assistive technology has altered the social and cultural context of educational environments.

These changes have also created opportunities for new partnerships among government, industry, educators, practitioners, children, and families. For example, educators have partnered with industry to ensure that the design of software programs meets the educational needs of a wide array of potential consumers. One of the most important outcomes of such partnerships is that they invigorate the concept of building healthy communities and developing community capacity to support people living with (and without) disabilities and restrictions; in other words, "partnerships involve the establishment of mutually beneficial relationships" (McBeth & Schweer, 2000, p. 76). Increased access to educational technology within schools enables all students, including those with special needs, to prepare to participate in an increasingly technologically dependent culture.

The Challenge

1. Read the case study of Wayne and complete the Client Profile and Task Analysis Form provided in Appendix J. Complete the form's sections on occupational history, interests, values, needs, performance patterns, and client factors. Identify the activity demands and contextual variables of his environments that currently challenge Wayne beyond his capabilities, and complete the required body structures and functions section on the form.

   To complete your analysis of Wayne's motor performance skills and sensory functions, answer the following questions:

   a. Why does Wayne use a power wheelchair for functional and community mobility? Why does he need a special seating system? Why do you think that the upright position of 90 degrees of hip flexion is Wayne's most functional sitting position?

   b. Why does Wayne use his left hand to push his right arm toward the numeric or function keys or lean his entire trunk to the right in an effort to reach the keys at the outer borders of his conventional keyboard? Why is he unable to return to a vertical position if he leans too far to the right or left?

c. Why is Wayne still able to control the joystick on his power wheelchair?

2. Wayne has collaborated with you in determining that one goal of intervention is to help him find a way to independently operate his computer. Using information from the case study and your task analysis, define the goals and objectives for intervention (a sample format is provided in Appendix K).

3. Become familiar with the process of setting up computers and peripheral devices.

   a. Set up and operate a computer with a miniature or expanded keyboard.

   b. Set up and operate a computer using a single switch with an interface device. Practice using the scanning and Morse code access methods.

   c. Use a mounting system such as the Mighty Mount (Tash International Inc.), Universal Table Mount (Tash International Inc.), Slim Armstrong™ (AbleNet Inc.), or Universal Mount (AbleNet Inc.) to set up a switch so that it can be controlled with the client's chin.

4. Would repositioning the keyboard on the table or a lap tray affect Wayne's independence and success in accessing the function and numeric keys? How could you reposition the keyboard? You have repositioned the keyboard so that it is closer to Wayne, but he is still unable to reach all of the function and numeric keys. What low-technology assistive devices would you consider trying with Wayne? What high-technology assistive devices would you consider trying? Review the different low- and high-technology assistive devices that are commercially available through catalogs and Web sites.

5. Twenty-four percent of people with disabilities have a computer at home, compared to 52 percent of nondisabled people, and 11 percent have access to the Internet at home, compared to 30 percent of nondisabled people. As an occupational therapy practitioner, how might you contribute to promoting participation in computer-based occupations among the populations who do not have access?

6. In 1998 Congress passed the Assistive Technology Act to assist states in maintaining and strengthening a permanent comprehensive statewide program of technology-related assistance for persons of all ages with disabilities. The act calls for the design of programs to (among other things) increase the availability of funding for, access to, and provision of assistive technology devices and services. Consider how occupational therapy practitioners can contribute with others to implement Title I of the act, which requires states and territories to conduct the following activities:

   a. Support a public awareness program designed to provide information on the availability and benefits of assistive technology devices and services.

   b. Promote interagency coordination that improves access to assistive technology devices and services for persons of all ages with disabilities.

   c. Provide technical assistance and training toward the development and implementation of laws, regulations, policies, practices, procedures, or organizational structures that promote access to assistive technology devices and services.

   d. Provide outreach support to statewide community-based organizations that provide assistive devices or services to persons with disabilities, including persons from underrepresented and rural populations, or assist them in using assistive technology devices and services.

7. U.S. culture has become increasingly dependent on technology. How has the "technology revolution"

   • altered social demands and expectations (i.e., activity demands)?

   • changed the cultural context of schools, workplaces, and homes?

   • affected activity demands in the education, work, and leisure occupations?

- increased opportunities for people to participate in education and work?
- influenced the temporal contexts of people?

8. Consider the potential influence of current and emerging technologies on the creation of virtual environments and how virtual contexts may support or hinder engagement in occupations. Appendix D provides a definition of virtual contexts. ▪

Learning Resources

AbleNet: www.ablenetinc.com

Alliance for Technology Access: www.ataccess.org

Americans With Disabilities Act: www.ada.org

Assistive Technology Act: www.resna.org/ata

Assistive Technology Training Online Project: www.atto.buffalo.edu

Center for Applied Special Technology: www.cast.org

Closing the Gap: Computer Technology in Special Education and Rehabilitation: www.closingthegap.com

Individuals With Disabilities Education Act: www.ideapractices.org, www.ed.gov/offices/OSERS/Policy/IDEA/the_law.html

Network of Regional Technology in Education Consortia: www.rtec.org

President's Commission on Excellence in Special Education: www.ed.gov/inits/commissionsboards/whspecialeducation

Rehabilitation Act: www.ed.gov/offices/OSERS/RSA

Rehabilitation Engineering and Rehabilitation Society of North America: www.resna.org

Tash International Inc.: www.tashinc.com

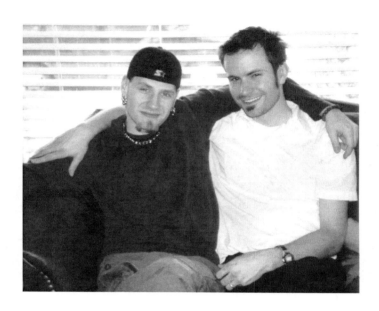

CHAPTER 12

Social Participation as Occupation

Understanding the interplay of development and contextual factors is important to assessing risk and opportunity in adolescent development and in planning appropriate intervention.

—Kenny, 1996, p. 476

CHAPTER OBJECTIVES

- To describe the use of task analysis in evaluation and intervention to develop strategies that enable adolescents to develop performance skills and patterns for social participation.
- To guide the completion of an occupational profile and a task analysis of a client that identifies performance skills and patterns, contexts, and client factors that affect adaptation; the establishment of client goals and objectives; and a group intervention plan.
- To describe the role of occupational therapy practitioners in promoting adolescent mental health.

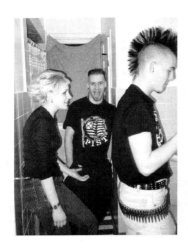

Social Participation as Occupation

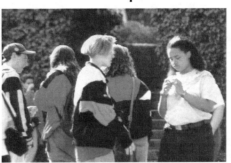

A dolescence, which occurs in the second decade of the life span, is a phase of growth and development marked by transitional changes in areas of occupation (e.g., social participation), performance skills (e.g., process skills), performance patterns (e.g., roles), and client factors (e.g., reproductive and mental functions). Adolescence is a time when there is a rapid expansion of roles. Children have several roles (e.g., son, daughter, sister, brother, friend), but adolescents take on new and complex roles (e.g., boyfriend, girlfriend, lover, employee, manager, parent), and their relationships with family, peers, and friends undergo changes. Although the family continues to be important and influential, peers may have a more powerful influence on an adolescent's decision making and problem solving (Steinberg, 1998).

Engagement in Social Participation

Social participation is the dimension of the occupational therapy domain that relates to "organized patterns of behavior that are characteristic and expected of an individual or an individual interacting with others within a given social system" (American Occupational Therapy Association [AOTA], 2002, p. 621; see also Mosey, 1996).

The components of social participation for adolescents include both successful interaction with family, peers, and friends and activities at the community level within neighborhoods, organizations, work, and school.

"It is important to recognize the coherence or continuity in development across life stages, as well as the factors that contribute to discontinuity. Understanding the interplay of developmental and contextual factors is important to assessing risk and opportunity in adolescent development and in planning appropriate interventions" (Kenny, 1996, p. 476). Personal contexts shift during adolescence. To begin with, adolescents experience change in the way they view themselves in relation to their capacity to function independently. Being independent is more than feeling independent; it means that one must be able to make one's own decisions and select a sensible course of action (Steinberg, 1998). Continued development of self-identity is linked to the sense of autonomy achieved through independence.

Developmental (i.e., client) and contextual (i.e., personal and environment) factors can provide opportunities for adolescents to expand and enhance their social participation, but they can also place adolescents at risk for ill health and dysfunctional behavior. The components of a successful transition to adulthood include moving from dependency and reliance on others to achieving economic self-sufficiency, establishing a home away from parents, attaining personal autonomy, and developing a personally satisfying lifestyle (Gorski & Miyake, 1985).

The interaction of persons, environments, and occupations is complex in the adolescent phase and is commonly perceived as perplexing. Adolescents undergo rapid changes in client factors, particularly in the areas of reproductive and mental functions. During the first few years of adolescence, people undergo biological transformations associated with puberty and become capable of reproduction. The physical changes in facial and other features related to puberty, coupled with the responsibilities associated with the ability to procreate, require adolescents to adjust to new life circumstances in a short time. One adaptation that can enhance well-being at this stage of life is to become comfortable with a changing experience of self and time in relation to body image, self-concept, and self-esteem. This ability to adjust and adapt is linked to the maturation of mental functions.

Maturation of mental functions in early adolescence is associated with a cognitive transition from concrete thinking, which is limited to what is "real" and "here and now" to higher-level, abstract thinking that involves the ability to think hypothetically and to observe reality as a backdrop for what is possible. As the adolescent moves into young adulthood, he or she uses higher-level thinking in constructing prospects for his or her (and society's) future. The adolescent can apply advanced reasoning to understand social situations and consider ideological concepts, alternative courses of action, and the consequences of choices and decisions. Indeed, as adolescents mature, they become better able to apply the mental functions of judgment, problem solving, reason, and logic to address challenging social circumstances and life situations. Newly formed cognitive and psychological attributes allow the

adolescent to interact with others, establish and maintain friendships and kinship bonds, cope with challenging situations, and manage his or her own behavior (Case-Smith, 1996).

Adolescence is also marked by changes in performance skills and patterns related to sleep, temperament, personality and emotional stability, and energy and drive. Performance skills (e.g., process skills) expand in the areas of energy, knowledge, and adaptation. Communication and interaction skills mature as adolescents learn new ways of communicating with others and begin to seek and establish intimate relationships. For example, adolescents learn new ways of interacting nonverbally with others (i.e. physicality). The importance of interactions between physical and mental functions is portrayed in adolescence. For example, the biological transformations associated with puberty (body structures) accompany changes in adolescents' sense of body (body functions), and communication and interaction performance skills (e.g., physicality) develop in response to increasingly complex occupations (social participation) and more challenging contexts (e.g., social environments). Clearly, the dynamic interaction among adolescents, environments, and occupations promotes rapid growth and development and requires adaptation.

In adolescence, physical prowess supports the development of identity, and physical abilities lead to specialization in skills acquisition, which in turn directs potential vocational choices. Self-expression reflects the use of a variety of styles and skills to express thoughts, feelings, and needs. Formal operational thought is the highlight of adolescence. Adolescents can conceptualize complex material, use reasoning in problem solving, and evaluate relationships (Shortridge, 1989). Performance patterns consist of automatic habits and routines that support occupational performance and establish sequences within the context of everyday living (AOTA, 2002).

This chapter provides readers an opportunity to use task analysis in evaluation and intervention to address the social participation of two adolescents. Barb has a history of attention deficit hyperactivity disorder (ADHD) and substance abuse, and recently she attempted suicide. Alana has recently been diagnosed with a conduct disorder. Her history includes substance abuse and arrest for prostitution.

Adolescent Health and Wellness

"Generally speaking, most young people are able to negotiate the biological, cognitive, emotional, and social transitions of adolescence successfully" (Steinberg, 1998, p. 9). However, the develop-

mental transition from childhood to adulthood leaves some adolescents vulnerable to a range of problems (Carnegie Council on Adolescent Development, 1995). Population research suggests that the health and well-being of adolescents are increasingly challenged by deviant and unhealthy behaviors (U.S. Department of Health and Human Services [DHHS], 2000). For example, tobacco and substance abuse are increasing, as are rates of mental illness and suicide. Additionally, although 85 percent of adolescents abstain from sexual intercourse or use

CASE STUDY: BARB

Barb is 13 years old and lives at home with her parents. She is the oldest of four children. Barb's mother and father are chronically underemployed and drink alcohol habitually. The family's struggle with poverty has depleted their emotional and psychological energy. Barb's mother vents frustration by constantly complaining to her husband that he should be working and by telling Barb that she is lazy and cannot do anything right. When Barb's parents binge drink, they leave her alone at home to care for her siblings. It is not unusual for them to be absent from the home throughout an entire night. Barb's father is easily frustrated, and he yells constantly at his children and has hit his wife on occasion. Barb's mother is 32 years old and attractive, and tension between Barb and her mother has increased now that Barb has reached puberty and matured physically.

At age 7 years, Barb was diagnosed with attention deficit hyperactivity disorder (ADHD). Throughout her school years, she had pervasive

problems with learning, and tutoring made little difference to Barb's academic performance. By age 9 she had lost interest in school and most other activities. But she always has enjoyed listening to music alone in her bedroom. Indeed, Barb often retreats to her room as a method of coping with challenging situations. By age 10 she began to have suicidal thoughts and to act out at school. She was disruptive in the classroom, required one-to-one time with the teacher to stay on task, and fought with other children on the playground. The gap between her academic achievement and that of her peers increased each school year. At 12 years she began to smoke and use alcohol on a daily basis. By 13 years, drug, alcohol, and tobacco addictions were a predominant part of her life.

Barb was recently hospitalized for rehabilitation following a suicide attempt. She was just discharged and is being seen daily by Kelsey, an occupational therapy practitioner at ABC Adolescent Services Center. During an interview with Barb's mother,

she reported to Kelsey that Barb's typical response to frustration at home is to become physically aggressive by banging doors and pushing, pinching, or shoving her siblings. She apparently will not listen when her parents try to talk to her about school or homework, and she sometimes walks away without warning and goes to her bedroom. Her mother reports that Barb has lost interest in taking care of herself.

Barb admits feeling "worthless." She has been diagnosed with depression and appears incapacitated by her depressed mood, saying that she simply "does not care what happens any longer." She does not appear to have any insight into her addictive behaviors and vehemently insists that she could take or leave alcohol and drugs whenever she opted to do so. She denies that she becomes physically and verbally aggressive at school and at home when she is frustrated or angry. Barb indicates that she has no friends, although she admits that she would like to have a girlfriend. ■

CASE STUDY: ALANA

Alana is 15 years old and lives in an upper-middle-class home with her father and 12-year-old sister. She was recently diagnosed with a conduct disorder. Alana's parents divorced when she was 11 years old, and her father was granted custody of the children because of her mother's problems with substance abuse. Because Alana's father is a lawyer who works long hours on workdays, he has employed Marni to manage the girls and the household. He is very generous with the girls, and they have more than enough money to meet their leisure needs.

Over the past 2 years Alana's father has become increasingly concerned about her behavior. Alana often stays out late at night and becomes angry when he tries to curtail her absences from home. She is wearing increasingly provocative clothes. Marni has expressed concern that Alana has not eaten at home very often over the past year and is beginning to look very gaunt. Recently, Marni gave notice of her intent to quit work, stating that Alana had become too disruptive and was

being verbally abusive toward her and her sister.

Alana has an extended history of negative behavior. By age 8 years, Alana had become aggressive in her play with peers. As the years progressed, teachers were unable to foster goodwill between Alana and the other children. Eventually she became more and more socially isolated and had no close friends. Even though her mother was often self-absorbed, Alana relied on her for company outside of school. Mother and daughter would shop together frequently, and the two watched television together while her mother drank alcohol excessively. By age 11, Alana was drinking with her mother. At that point in her life Alana had become belligerent with all adults and was bullied by her peers. It was this behavior that led to her father's decision to obtain a divorce and seek custody of the girls.

Alana's loneliness became acute with her mother's absence from the family home. She experimented with hanging out with a group of street kids and found that they were more than willing to involve her in their activities.

She became quite popular because of her easy access to money to buy drugs and ability to sneak alcohol from her home. Her chemical dependency quickly progressed to cocaine addiction by the time she was 14 years old. At 15 she was arrested for prostitution and possession of drugs.

This crisis brought Alana to ABC Adolescent Services Center. After initial detoxification, Alana began to receive services on a daily basis from Kelsey, an occupational therapy practitioner. Kelsey was impressed with the level of participation of Alana's father and sister in her program, and she sees positive results in the changes in Alana's insight, attitude, and behavior. Preparation for discharge is the next stage in the intervention program. Arrangements have already been made for Alana to attend a private, all-girls school after her discharge and to continue to live in the family home. The school provides a small classroom setting and in-school counseling services. Alana's father has hired a new partner in his firm and intends to cut his workload to be home with the girls in the morning and after school. ■

condoms if they are sexually active, roughly 1 million teenage girls have unintentional pregnancies each year. Furthermore, despite evidence that regular physical activity throughout life is important for maintaining a healthy body, enhancing psychological well-being, and preventing premature death, only two thirds of adolescents engage in the recommended amount of physical activity. Among children and adolescents ages 6 to 19 years, 11 percent are overweight or obese (DHHS, 2000). The leading causes of death

among adolescents in the United States are unintentional injuries, homicide, and suicide. Over the past two decades, suicidal behavior, criminal activity, antisocial patterns, low achievement, eating disorders, and depression have increased substantially among adolescents (Rutters, 1995; Zahn-Waxler, 1996).

Mental health, tobacco use, substance abuse, violence, and responsible sexual behavior are five of the 10 leading public health concerns in the United States; *Healthy People 2010* describes the nation's vision, goals, and objectives for improving health. Approximately 20 percent of the U.S. population is affected by mental illness during a given year, and depression is the most common disorder. Major depression is the leading cause of disability and is associated with more than two thirds of suicides each year (DHHS, 2000). Depression in adolescence is often masked as behavior disorders or delinquency (Florey, 1998). Symptoms include diminished interest or loss of pleasure in most activities, mood changes (e.g, crankiness, sadness, feelings of hopelessness), sleep difficulties, irritability, social withdrawal, and suicidal ideation or attempts (Florey, 1998).

Depression is complex and is generally interrelated with comorbid psychosocial problems; for example, dysfunctional or maladaptive process skills and communication and interaction skills may lower a person's capacity to cope with challenging life situations. Wilcock (1998) noted, "If individuals are under- or overstressed in the use of emotional, intellectual, or spiritual capacities because of physiological, environmental, or social factors, or because of occupational deprivation, alienation, or imbalance, health and well-being may be undermined" (p. 102). Duggal (2000) found that 97 percent of adolescents with a depressive disorder reported an experience of a severe negative life event either in preadolescence or during adolescence (e.g., family crisis, parental health issues, educational problems, difficulty with peer relationships). Suicidal behavior and substance dependence, two of society's most serious problems, are often comorbid with depressive disorders, psychological distress, or disruption in the family system (Cavaiola, 1999).

On the basis of extensive research, DHHS (2000) recently asserted that "cigarette smoking is the single most preventable cause of disease and death in the United States" and "results in more deaths each year…than AIDS, alcohol, cocaine, heroin, homicide, suicide, motor vehicle crashes, and fires—combined" (p. 30). In 1997, 36 percent of adolescents smoked, reflecting an increase in smoking among students in grades 9 through 12 during the 1990s. Every day an estimated 3,000 young people start smoking, and almost half of adolescents who continue to smoke regularly will eventually die from smoking-related illness (DHHS, 2000).

DHHS (2000) has also associated alcohol and illicit drug use with other serious problems, including violence, injury, and HIV infection. In 1997, 77 percent of adolescents ages 12 to 17 years reported being alcohol or drug free in the preceding month, but 21 percent reported drinking alcohol, 8 percent reported binge drinking, and 10 percent reported using illicit drugs.

ADHD is one of the most common disorders in adolescence, and health conditions associated with ADHD include depression and social isolation. Typically a child is diagnosed before age 7 years, and characteristics of inattentiveness and hyperactivity–impulsivity continue in full or residual form into adolescence and adulthood (Hansen, 1999). Children diagnosed with ADHD experience several developmental hardships by the time they reach adolescence. They frequently have difficulty engaging in education occupations and often have poor grades and drop out of school (Hansen, 1999). Persons who have not completed high school may be disadvantaged in seeking, attaining, and maintaining desired employment in a competitive marketplace. In addition, the social sequela of ADHD may seriously limit social participation. Adolescents with maladaptive behavior associated with ADHD are at risk for social isolation; aggressive behavior and poor social skills may limit peer relationships to brief interactions, and impulsivity often excludes adolescents from healthy social networks. Adolescents with ADHD may exhibit delinquent and antisocial behavior to seek acceptance by unconventional social groups.

Using Task Analysis to Promote Health Among Adolescents

Occupational therapy services with adolescents who have activity limitations and participation restrictions may be provided through schools, community agencies, hospitals, outpatient clinical settings, or other institutional settings. Occupational therapy practitioners use task analysis as an evaluation and intervention tool to analyze the dynamic interaction among adolescents, their environments, and their occupations and to identify factors that support or hinder participation in healthy life situations. Adolescents experiencing the consequences of maladjustment can benefit from occupational therapy when this maladjustment affects engagement in occupations (e.g., social participation), participation in contexts, role competency, quality of life, and healthy lifestyles.

During the evaluation phase, occupational therapy practitioners interview adolescent clients; these clients are able to be reflective and to articulate their interests, needs, and priorities. Adolescent (and adult) clients often tell stories about their lives, and these narratives assist practitioners in understanding mental health issues and areas of concern (Lewin & Reed, 1998; Neistadt, 1998; Wilcock, 1998). Each piece of information offered in an interview may be linked to an explanation of behavior or lead to collaborative solutions (Dunn, 2000; Kielhofner, 1995; Lewin & Reed, 1998). The interviewer both listens for information and seeks to appreciate the spirit of the communication. Skilled interviewers artfully phrase open-ended questions and consider the timing of their asking (Davis, 1989; Dunn, 2000). Henry (1998) noted that an important factor to consider during an interview is "the inherent power imbalance in the relationship between the child and an adult interviewer" (p. 158); therefore, establishing rapport and trust is critical to the therapeutic relationship.

Interpersonal relationships that involve therapeutic use of self, interpersonal rapport, and collaboration characterize the helping relationship and are an essential feature of practice (AOTA, 1995; Lewin & Reed, 1998; Mosey, 1986; Wilcock, 1998). The therapeutic relationship is "one of the most important and powerful tools in client-centered intervention" because the emo-

tional atmosphere of therapy influences client expectations, attitude, and trust. This relationship transforms the adolescent's behavior from "constructive dependency" to "functional autonomy" (Canadian Association of Occupational Therapists [CAOT], 1991, p. 61). The body of an interview is guided by the use of key questions that address the individual's reason for seeking intervention, including his or her perception of the problems; issues or challenges that are affecting performance; and the characteristics of the problem, issue, or challenge within the contexts of everyday living.

The occupational therapy profession embraces the belief that occupational engagement in a range of activities allows persons "to be creative and adventurous as they experience all human emotions, explore, and adapt appropriately and without disruption to meet their life needs" (Wilcock, 1998, p. 103). Use of purposeful activities is what separates occupational therapy from the verbal therapies (CAOT, 1993; Wilcock, 1998). Active engagement in purposeful activity is a catalyst in the development of self and in the fulfillment of social membership and can be "understood as motivation toward achieving a sense of competence, self-reliance, social role learning, and societal contribution" (AOTA, 1995a, p. 1021). Occupational therapy practitioners select a purposeful activity for use in intervention after determining whether an individual or group project, craft, or game motivates and fulfills clients' psychosocial and psychological needs. "Congruence between the characteristics of an activity and the biopsychosocial characteristics of the person" qualify an activity as purposeful (AOTA, 1995a, p. 1021; Fidler, 1981).

Occupations provide a "mechanism for social interaction and societal development and growth, forming the foundation of community, local, and national identity, because individuals not only engage in separate pursuits, they are able to plan and execute group activity" (Wilcock, 1998, p. 25). Small task groups are an occupational therapy intervention that provides both a therapeutic activity and a social context designed to induce changes in individual members. Such groups are broadly classified by purpose: (a) therapeutic, (b) peer support, (c) focus or study, and (d) consultation and supervision (Schwartzberg, 1998, p. 121). The activity, the social milieu, and group dynamics can all be structured to replicate the daily living challenges participants encounter in their natural social environments (Davidson, 1991). The verbal and nonverbal interactive group process provides motivation, support, and feedback to reinforce learning and promote adaptation. Practitioners who lead groups must be flexible, offer appropriate and sincere encouragement, possess interpersonal sensitivity, teach new skills, share information, and provide guidance (Gorski & Miyake, 1985).

Social participation is a central occupation for adolescents. Peer groups provide socialization opportunities and a venue for learning new skills and behaviors (Donohue & Greer, 2000). Such groups are process oriented and generally aimed at changing participants' behavior (Kielhofner, 1997; Schwartzberg, 1998). Group leaders choose tasks to establish or restore a skill or ability, to maintain or preserve performance capabilities, and to develop compensatory strategies and adaptive responses. Adolescents often have difficulty setting goals, both individually and in groups, most likely because the task is so abstract. Donohue and Greer (2000) suggested that "perhaps their peers jointly devalue goals in groups in which attendance is mandatory" (p. 168). One way to make goals seem less abstract and more binding is to have adolescent participants sign a contract. Peer support groups may function for that singular goal of providing support for adolescents, families, caregivers, and partners, often around a shared problem or disability. Peer support group facilitators most often use a structured dialogue or instructional format, and the larger the group, the less it is able to be process oriented.

Occupational therapy practitioners use a variety of group approaches. The following elements are common to productive group interventions:

- Group-centered activity with maximum involvement and motivation of each member

- Development of a group through a shared "doing" that provides realistic experiences to members in a supportive environment in which they can learn skills and modify behavior
- A temporal "flow" in task engagement
- Consistent support and feedback from leaders and members (Kielhofner, 1997; Schwartzberg, 1998).

The occupational therapy practitioner maintains group cohesion and individual goal direction by continuously observing the group; making in-progress adjustments to directions and task objectives; and engaging in therapeutic exchange with participants and the group as a whole through empathic communication, modeling behavior, and reality testing.

The Challenge

1. How did your childhood experience provide a foundation for your adolescence? What activities and occupations did you participate in and enjoy throughout adolescence? What characteristics and qualities of these activities promoted your personal and social development during adolescence?

2. Read "Position Paper: The Psychosocial Core of Occupational Therapy" (AOTA, 1995) and describe AOTA's perspective on the role of occupational therapy in addressing the psychosocial needs of clients.

3. Read the case studies of Barb and Alana and complete a Client Profile and Task Analysis Form for each of the girls. A blank copy of this form is provided in Appendix J. Complete the Client Profile, Performance Patterns, Performance Skills, Client Factors, and Contexts sections of the form. Use this client analysis to develop a purposeful activity and determine intervention strategies for use in a group context. Consider the following questions as you develop the occupational profiles for these clients:

   a. When you learn about Barb's and Alana's life stories, it is natural for you to evaluate their life circumstances in terms of your own personal values, beliefs, and paradigms. What are your comfort zones in discussing personal histories with clients when they include information about violence, substance abuse, mental illness, and prostitution? What must you do to shift the boundaries you have formed personally before conducting an interview with these two clients?

b. What interview tools might you use to explore these clients' social participation and identify issues in their performance skills and patterns?

4. Document specific, measurable, outcome-oriented goals and objectives for both clients (a sample format for writing client goals is provided in Appendix K). In practice, you would establish these goals in collaboration with the clients and in consultation with their parents.

5. Kelsey, an occupational therapy practitioner, completed an initial evaluation of Barb and Alana and wondered about the possibility of arranging for these two clients to receive services jointly in areas in which their goals were similar. She decided to schedule both adolescents to attend the same session and have them work together on an activity.

a. Why might Kelsey have elected to see these two clients together rather than individually?

b. What differences in the girls' characteristics must Kelsey consider when conducting group sessions with the two of them?

c. In what areas do the adolescents' performance skills and patterns have the potential to positively or negatively influence the other?

6. Use your understanding of Barb's and Alana's occupational performance profiles to select an appropriate purposeful activity for the group session. Ensure that the selected activity addresses their goals, interests, values, and needs. The characteristics of purposeful activities are described in Appendix L. Should Barb and Alana be involved in the selection of a therapeutic activity? Provide a rationale.

7. Find a partner to engage in the activity you have selected and structured for this group. Take turns role-playing client and therapist. Role-playing provides insight into the therapeutic value of rapport and enables you to increase the accuracy of your analysis and develop your skills in client interaction.

8. Design a sequenced activity plan to provide services that will help these clients attain the goals and objectives you have set together.

9. How might occupational therapy practitioners work with other professionals to address factors within the family contexts that influence Barb's and Alana's adaptation?

10. In 2000 the U.S. Department of Health and Human Services outlined a comprehensive nationwide agenda to improve the health of the population. Because the research findings on the health of the nation's adolescents were cause for concern, many of the goals and objectives of this plan relate to adolescents. The *Healthy People 2010* agenda includes health goals, objectives, and indicators that are "grounded in science, built through public consensus, and designed to measure progress" (DHHS, 2000, p. 1). One of the target goals identified in this agenda is to

increase the proportion of middle, junior high, and senior high schools that provide school health education to prevent health problems in the following areas: unintentional injury; violence; suicide; tobacco use and addiction; alcohol and other drug use; unintended pregnancy, HIV/AIDS, and STD infection; unhealthy dietary patterns; inadequate physical activity; and environmental health. (http://www.healthypeople.gov/document/html/objectives/07-02.htm)

How might an occupational therapy practitioner provide services or resources to community organizations promoting the development of health initiatives for adolescents? ◼

Learning Resources

Addiction Resource Guide: www.addictionresourceguide.com

Attention Deficit Disorder Association: www.add.org

Depression and Related Affective Disorders Association: www.drada.com

Drug and Alcohol Treatment Intervention Global Network: www.ddrugnet.net

Mayo Clinic: www.mayoclinic.com/findinformation/diseasesandconditions

The National Council on Alcoholism and Drug Dependence: www.ncadd.org

National Institute of Mental Health: www.nimh.nih.gov

Office of Special Education: http://curry.edschool.virginia.edu

Psychiatry Matters: www.psychiatrymatters.md

Teen Risk Resource Center: www.teenrisk.com

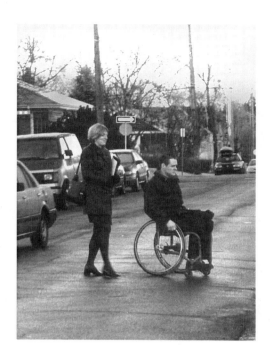

CHAPTER 13

Maintaining Meaningful Lifestyles

Disability is a natural part of the human experience and in no way diminishes the right of individuals to live independently; enjoy self-determination and make choices; benefit from an education; pursue meaningful careers; and enjoy full inclusion and integration into the economic, political, social, cultural, and educational mainstream of society.

—Assistive Technology Act, 1998

CHAPTER OBJECTIVES
- To describe the use of task analysis in evaluation and intervention with adults to determine and optimize the degree of fit between the client's current and desired engagement and participation in areas of occupation.
- To describe how occupational therapy practitioners use task analysis to match community resources, agencies, and social support systems to the needs of the persons who have activity limitations and participation restrictions.

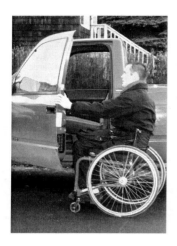

Maintaining Meaningful Lifestyles

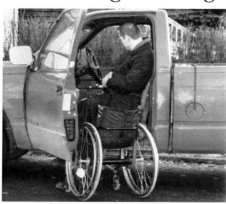

Adulthood represents an achieved state of maturity. As a phase of development, adulthood typically begins with enhanced personal freedom, choice, and responsibility as one learns to care for oneself and others emotionally, spiritually, physically, and financially. "Some of the changes [that occur throughout adulthood] are externally recognizable as the person passes through a series of steps, crises or transitions: marriage or divorce, starting a family, changing jobs, and bidding farewell to grown children" (Kielhofner, 1995, p. 446).

Adulthood is a time for choosing a lifestyle and assuming new and complex roles: friend, lover, spouse, student, colleague, boss, worker, breadwinner, parent, citizen, and so forth. Roles organize behavior, communicate expectations, and evolve across the life span. Roles add pleasure and enjoyment to life, contribute to achievement, and help maintain the self and family life (Christiansen & Baum, 1991; Kielhofner, 1995; Watson, 1997). One's identity as an adult is often shaped by the roles one assumes in society. These roles are influenced by environmental and personal contexts. Competency in the role of worker is a primary expectation of adults in most societies. Role competence is an occupational therapy outcome (see

Figure 1.1; American Occupational Therapy Association [AOTA], 2002).

Adulthood is always a time of personal growth. A person's identity, self-concept, and life plans evolve and are influenced by unpredictable events. When a person's ability to participate in meaningful occupations is restricted, his or her life plans must undergo a transformation (Frank, 1996a; Polkinghorne, 1996). People are holistic entities, and injury, impairment, or underdevelopment in one area may affect a person's entire identity. Likewise, changes in a person's identity can influence the degree to which impairments limit participation in occupations (Polkinghorne, 1996).

Adaptation refers to the adjustments persons make to enhance their ability to survive and thrive in the context of unforeseen circumstances. Adaptive attitudes and skills help people master life challenges and actualize their potential. Adaptation requires and is the result of changes in persons and their desired tasks and roles as well as personal and environmental contexts (AOTA, 1993; Mosey, 1986). To adapt, people must take an active role in responding to specific contextual demands (King, 1978). Adaptation is also an occupational therapy outcome (see Figure 1.1; AOTA, 2002).

Activity Limitations and Participation Restrictions

Traumatic injuries such as amputations, spinal cord injuries, and brain injuries usually cause permanent, irreversible impairments that alter a person's ability to participate in his or her customary roles and occupations. Impairments and activity limitations, however, need not negatively affect the client's spirit, belief in personal causation, perceived self-efficacy, self-concept, or sense of mastery over life events. *Personal causation* refers to a person's belief in his or her abilities, perception of control over behavior and outcomes, and expectation of success in future endeavors (Kielhofner, 1985). Autonomy is linked with a sense of *self-efficacy*, which is an individual's judgment of his or her capacity to use existing skills to attain certain levels of performance (Kielhofner, 1995). *Self-concept* refers to the value that the person places on the physical, emotional, and sexual self (AOTA, 1994b). When a permanent impairment suddenly alters a client's ability to engage in occupations and participate in customary contexts, he or she is unable to rely on familiar performance patterns to continue in customary roles. Familiar behaviors and customary roles give people a sense of being a part of their social community and culture. Adaptation skills are required to regain a sense of competency in customary roles and participation in the contexts of their community and culture.

As illustrated in the Occupational Therapy Services Model (described in chapter 1), role competence, adaptation, and engagement in occupations are linked. Occupational therapy practitioners combine their understanding of a client's impairments, activity limitations, participation restrictions, and premorbid lifestyle with knowledge gained from experience in working with other clients who have similar disabilities to construct an image of their client's future potential. Clients guide the intervention process through their participation in the construction, revision, and realization of a "possible and desirable future" (Mattingly & Flemming, 1994, p. 241). With experience, practitioners are able to make increasingly accurate predictions about their clients' potential functional status. Practitioners direct intervention toward enabling clients to envision and re-establish a satisfying lifestyle by establishing, reconstructing, and controlling their patterns of occupation. In this way, occupational therapy practitioners facilitate adaptation (AOTA, 1994b). Occupational therapy practitioners design intervention to promote engagement and participation in desired occupations and roles and enhance clients' participation in activities for which they have high interest but low satisfaction (Yerxa & Baum, 1986).

The compensatory or adaptation approach to intervention involves finding ways for the client to revise activity demands and contexts to support his or her participation in natural settings (AOTA, 2002). To successfully adapt, the client must appraise his or her values and goals and work toward attainment of personal, social, and vocational plans (Versluys, 1995). Occupational therapy practitioners working with clients with long-standing impairments collaborate with the clients to define outcome goals and objectives in all areas of occupation: basic and instrumental activities of daily living, education, work, play, leisure, and social participation.

The initial stages of recovery are usually associated with low levels of energy and endurance, and basic activities of daily living (BADL) usually are addressed first. In addition, clients' dignity and self-esteem often depend on their doing or directing their own self-care. Participation in work, play, leisure, and social occupations commences when the client has regained enough stamina. Activity limitations in these areas result in loss of opportunity to participate in intrinsically motivating and highly rewarding occupations. For example, loss of choice in play and leisure pursuits may affect volition and individuality (Bundy, 1993). Conversely, participation in sports may increase sense of mastery, self-esteem, adjustment to loss, social interaction, and level of

CASE STUDY: LAURIE

Laurie is a 40-year-old married woman who was the sole occupant in a single-vehicle automobile accident. She was driving home from a party where she had been drinking wine all evening. Laurie was always busy throughout December with promotional parties and obligatory engagements; the business of marketing and advertising in the fashion industry is very competitive, and visibility, reputation, and consistency in performance were Laurie's secrets to success.

Laurie began her career as a fashion model at age 14. By the time she was in her early 20s, she had posed on the cover of several national women's magazines. In her teens and early 20s she worked freelance selling fashion illustrations but never made enough money to support her desired lifestyle. She was married at age 25 to a successful interior designer and began a college program in journalism and photography with a minor in art history shortly thereafter. Immediately after graduation Laurie worked as a freelance journalist writing articles on women's apparel and accessories. As she gained more experience, she began publishing photographs to accompany her articles. Three years after graduation, Laurie became the owner and chief executive officer of ABC Marketing, combining her knowledge of fashion and skills as a writer and photographer. The firm has three employees, profits have soared, and Laurie's family has come to depend on her income.

After the accident Laurie received rehabilitation services to recover from a left upper-limb above-elbow amputation, extensive internal injuries, and multiple abrasions to her face and upper body. Occupational therapy intervention was directed primarily toward Laurie's learning to use a prosthesis with her dominant left arm. By the time she was discharged, Laurie was able to use her prosthesis to independently dress herself and cook a meal. Twelve months following her accident, Laurie visited her family physician at the request of her husband. The doctor prescribed antidepressant medication. Two weeks later, on her 40th birthday, Laurie attempted suicide by ingesting over-the-counter sleeping pills and was admitted to the hospital.

During the occupational therapy evaluation, Laurie was quiet and slow to respond to questions. She wore a long-sleeved shirt and sweatpants, held her left upper arm with her right hand, and did not have her prosthesis. Laurie indicated that her interest and energy levels were very low and that she would prefer to sleep. Although prompted to discuss her personal goals, Laurie avoided this request and did not respond. She indicated that she intended to return to work. Although she had sustained her business by working out of her home for 2 months after her accident, Laurie had not worked since then. She described her marriage as turbulent and her husband and 14-year-old daughter as the only "constants" in her life. Laurie suggested that her relationship with her husband was "strained" and made the following observations: "He probably is just not attracted to me anymore." "I don't blame him…look at me; I'm useless." "I often wonder why he stays with me." "I always went to parties alone, and he would stay at home with our daughter." "He always hated my friends." "I know they need me to work, but I just can't do it. Things won't change." "I just don't feel like seeing anyone." ■

---

physical fitness for a person with a disability (Pasek & Schkade, 1996; Stotts, 1986; Taylor & McGruder, 1996; Valliant, Bezzubyk, Daley, & Asu, 1985). Whereas some clients are initially interested in returning to their former work, play, and leisure occupations, others may benefit from being introduced to novel activities and occupations to assist in the construction of a new identity and sense of self (Taylor & McGruder, 1996). The role of occupational therapy practitioners who work with people with long-term impairments, therefore, is to restructure activity demands, alter environmental contexts, teach new methods, introduce new options, and facilitate adaptation.

The Challenge

Read one or more of the case studies of Laurie, Jeff, and Rena, and complete the questions pertaining to each.

Work and Social Participation: Laurie

1. Read the case about Laurie and complete the Client Profile and Task Analysis Form provided in Appendix J. Complete the Client Profile, Performance Patterns, Performance Skills, Client Factors, and Contexts sections of the form.

2. What are your perceptions of Laurie's sense of personal causation, perceived self-efficacy, and self-concept? Consider the long-term potential for a person with an above-elbow amputation in terms of performance skills and participation in occupations. Has Laurie lived up to this potential? If not, what might be the reasons? Do you think Laurie's depression might be caused by or related to the accident? How might you determine the answers to these important questions?

3. Use your understanding of Laurie's premorbid lifestyle, values and beliefs, and knowledge of the impact of her impairments to construct an image of her potential and occupational possibilities. This "possible and desirable future" for clients gives therapists a starting point and guides intervention (Mattingly & Flemming, 1994, p. 241).

4. Identify and set priorities. Document some specific, measurable, outcome-oriented goals and objectives for Laurie (see Appendix K). In practice, you would establish these goals and objectives in consultation with Laurie and her family, and together you would modify them once Laurie is prepared to work more collaboratively with the intervention team.

5. Develop an initial intervention plan by selecting an area of occupation identified in the client goals. Select and design a purposeful activity for use with Laurie during a 30-minute session. Consider designing an intervention plan for a group session that incorporates Laurie's goals with those of the others who have similar goals. Purposeful activities are therapeutic when they are relevant, meaningful, and goal directed and encourage mastery and feelings of competence

(AOTA, 1993). Direct an activity toward having Laurie be more active in the construction of a life plan and, therefore, in the identification of her own long-term goals and intervention objectives. The following learning resources assist you with this challenge: Gage (1992); Gage and Polatajko (1994); Helfrich and Kielhofner (1994); Helfrich, Kielhofner, and Mattingly (1994); Polkinghorne (1996); and Price-Lankey and Cashman (1996).

6. Among persons living in the community, those with disabilities are twice as likely to live alone as those who do not have disabilities (LaPlante, Carlson, Kaye, & Bradsher, 1996). As of 1994, persons with disabilities were also less likely to socialize with close friends, relatives, or neighbors; go to a movie; eat at a restaurant; attend a live music performance; or attend a church or synagogue. In fact, comparisons with a similar 1986 poll show that the level of social participation of people with disabilities has remained unchanged (Kaye, 1998). As an occupational therapy practitioner, how might you contribute to promoting participation and health among this population? What social support groups in your city or state might be a resource in the establishment of health-promoting activities and events in communities?

Play, Leisure, and Social Participation: Jeff

1. Read the case study of Jeff and complete the Client Profile, Performance Patterns, Performance Skills, Client Factors, and Contexts sections of the Client Profile and Task Analysis Form provided in Appendix J.

2. Why have initial therapy sessions focused on engagement in activities to enhance the motor performance skills affected by the motor functions of endurance, postural stability, and upper-extremity strength? Why might Jeff prefer to put on his undergarments, pants, and shirt while sitting on the bed? Why might Jeff be slow at tying his shoes? Consider the activity demands of these activities.

CASE STUDY: JEFF

Jeff is a 32-year-old single man who sustained a midthoracic, complete spinal cord injury and a mild traumatic brain injury during a recent motor vehicle accident. He plans to return to his job as a sports commentator and has expressed an interest in participating in wheelchair sports. Jeff is fond of baseball, basketball, football, tennis, rugby, fishing, water sports, and camping. Initial therapy sessions on the rehabilitation unit focus on engagement in activities to build endurance, enhance postural stability, increase upper-extremity strength, and learn new methods of performing basic activities of daily living (BADL).

Although Jeff appears to have mild visual–perceptual and short-term memory problems, results of the assessment suggest that his initial lack of independence in BADL may be due primarily to paralysis.

After the first few weeks of intervention, Jeff gained independence in dressing, personal care, and bathing. Jeff can put his undergarments, pants, and shirt on and take them off while sitting in bed. Jeff puts on his shoes while sitting in his wheelchair and is quite slow tying his shoelaces. He requires standby assistance to ensure that he safely transfers to a raised toilet seat and a tub bench seat. His occupational therapy practitioner predicts that

he will eventually transfer independently to a regular-height toilet seat and that he may always require some type of bath seat.

Jeff appears to be very goal directed and frequently verbalizes his commitment to returning to his previous lifestyle. He has not expressed any other feelings to his occupational therapy practitioner about his injury and does not speak much with the other patients in the hospital. Jeff's immediate family does not live nearby. His girlfriend visits regularly and is a physical therapist. Two other people with spinal cord injuries are on the rehabilitation unit at this time. ∎

3. Why were a raised toilet seat, bath bench seat, and wheelchair used to alter the physical context to promote Jeff's participation in bathing and functional mobility? Why did the occupational therapy practitioner predict that Jeff would continue to require some type of bath seat?

4. Use your understanding of Jeff's premorbid lifestyle and knowledge of the impact of his impairment to construct an image of his future potential and occupational possibilities.

   a. Do you think Jeff will be able to become independent in basic and instrumental activities of daily living? Explain and justify your impressions. Identify potential activity demands and contextual variables that might limit independence in this area. Identify and describe potential intervention strategies.

   b. Do you think that Jeff will be able to return to work as a sports commentator? Use the Client Profile and Task Analysis Form to assist you in this determination. Complete the Activity Demands section to profile the tasks in a typical workday. Then complete the Activity Demands and Client Factors section and compare the information in the Level of Demand and Level of Impairment columns. Consider the context of the workplace: Is there a match or fit among Jeff's performance capabilities, the activity demands of this job, and contextual factors? Explain and justify your impressions. Identify potential activity demands, physical contexts, performance limitations, and employment barriers that might limit Jeff's engagement in his customary work occupation.

   Jeff has collaborated with you to define goals and objectives for his rehabilitation, and one of his goals is to return to work. Write three short-term objectives to address this goal (a sample format is provided in Appendix K). Identify and describe potential intervention strategies. Appendix G lists approaches to intervention that you could consider. Is Jeff's employer required to make reasonable accommodations for his new disability? What type of accommodations may be necessary?

c. Do you think that Jeff will be able to actively participate in the sports he is fond of? Select one of these sports and consider the activity demands required to participate. Use the Client Profile and Task Analysis Form to assist you in this analysis. Complete the Activity Demands section to profile the tasks involved in participating in this sport. Then complete the Activity Demands and Client Factors section and compare the information in the Level of Demand and Level of Impairment columns. Consider the performance contexts of participation. Is there a match among Jeff's performance capabilities, the activity demands of this sport, and contextual factors? Explain and justify your impressions. Identify potential activity demands, performance limitations, and contextual barriers that might limit Jeff's engagement in the sport.

Jeff has collaborated with you to define goals and objectives for his rehabilitation, and one of his goals is to participate in this sport. Write three short-term objectives to address this goal (a sample format is provided in Appendix K). Identify and describe potential intervention strategies and assistive devices. Appendix G lists approaches to intervention you could consider.

d. Do you think Jeff will be able to drive? Use the Client Profile and Task Analysis Form to assist you in this determination. Complete the Activity Demands section to profile the task of driving Jeff's two-door, medium-size car. Then complete the Activity Demands and Client Factors section and compare the information in the Level of Demand and Level of Impairment columns. Is there a match or fit among Jeff's performance capabilities, the activity demands of this task, and contextual factors? Explain and justify your impressions. Identify potential activity demands, performance limitations, and contextual barriers that might limit Jeff's engagement in this area of occupation.

e. You have determined that Jeff can drive, and one of Jeff's goals is to drive. Write three short-term objectives to address this goal (a sample format is provided in Appendix K). Identify and describe potential intervention strategies and assistive devices that might be considered. Appendix G lists approaches to intervention you could consider.

f. Design a 30-minute session with Jeff to address one or more of his goals and objectives.

g. Identify one local agency that organizes sport activities for persons with disabilities.

h. Identify assistive technology devices that enable persons with disabilities to participate in a sport or drive a car.

5. Roughly 2.2 million noninstitutionalized Americans older than age 15 use a wheelchair. Another 6.4 million use some other ambulatory aid such as a cane, crutches, or a walker (McNeil, 2001). As an occupational therapy practitioner, how might you contribute to promoting participation and health among these populations? Might political advocacy be a role for an occupational therapy practitioner? If so, what types of activities might this role entail?

Play, Leisure, and Social Participation: Rena

1. Read the case study of Rena and complete the Client Profile and Task Analysis Form provided in Appendix J. Complete the Client Profile, Performance Patterns, Performance Skills, Client Factors, and Contexts sections of the form.

2. Use your understanding of Rena's premorbid lifestyle, values and beliefs, and knowledge of the impact of her impairments to construct an image of her potential and occupational possibilities. Determining how a diagnosed impairment or condition influences present performance and levels of participation can help occupational therapist practitioners make accurate predictions about potential gains in functional levels (Mattingly & Flemming, 1994).

CASE STUDY: RENA

Rena is a 40-year-old mother who was just transferred to a rehabilitation unit for recovery from a right ischemic cerebrovascular accident (CVA); a cardiogenic embolus lodged in her middle cerebral artery 2 weeks ago. Rena's medical chart indicates a history of coronary artery disease, arrhythmias, cardiomegaly, and hypercholesterolemia. Two years ago Rena was admitted to ABC Medical Center with atrial fibrillation. An echocardiogram showed a dilated aortic root, and a subsequent CT scan of the chest confirmed the diagnosis.

Rena is a divorced parent of two children: Jacob (11 years old) and Jason (7 years old). She does not have many close friends but has been dating Benjamin for 8 months. The children's grandmother is caring for them until their mother returns home from rehabilitation. Before her admission to the hospital, Rena worked full-time as a librarian at the elementary school

her children attend. She and her kids ride the school bus together each morning. Rena has gained a reputation for her literary, art, history, and poetry exhibitions, and the school's teachers are very fond of her. Rena enjoys homemaking and occasionally sews clothes for her children. She also had attended a continuing education course one night per week on advanced computer word processing. Jacob and Jason play baseball three nights a week and spend very little time at home on the weekends. They spend most of their spare time outdoors watching or participating in neighborhood baseball and basketball games. Rena is known on the boys' baseball team for her great hamburgers and chocolate chip cookies.

Rena, Jacob, and Jason live in a first-floor, two-bedroom apartment with a 6-in. step at the building entrance. Jacob has provided a graphic illustration of the layout of Rena's bedroom (Figure 13.1), the family's

kitchen (Figure 13.2), and the bathroom (Figure 13.3). The laundry room is located on the same floor as the apartment and has a 2-in. step at the doorway. The grocery store is four blocks away. Their neighborhood has a strong social network, but Rena indicates that she prefers not to "get involved" and doesn't like to "depend on anyone."

Rena's physiatrist estimates that she will require 4 more weeks of inpatient services. The physical therapist expects Rena eventually to walk short distances with a rolling walker and to use a manual wheelchair for community mobility. The admission note indicates that Rena had a flaccid left trunk and upper and lower extremities, left unilateral sensory loss in her upper limb more than in her lower limb, left ptosis, perceptual and cognitive deficits, and decreased attention. The occupational therapy evaluation is almost complete and you, as the occupational therapy

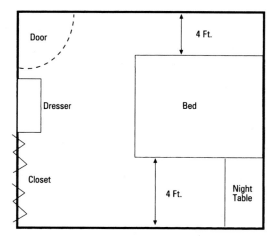

Figure 13.1. Rena's son's drawing of her bedroom.

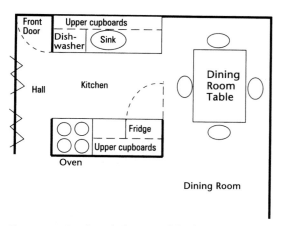

Figure 13.2. Rena's son's drawing of the family kitchen.

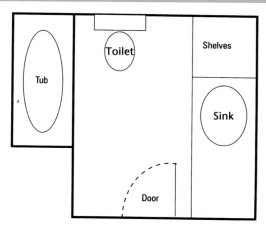

Figure 13.3. Rena's son's drawing of her bathroom.

practitioner, must assist the rehabilitation team in preparing Rena for discharge. Rena does not have any cardiac precautions at this time.

During the initial interview, Rena expresses her commitment to care for her two children: "Although they can help me out around the apartment, I don't want them to have to take care of me." "Sure I love my job, but my children come first." Rena is fiercely motivated to regain her independence and fully intends to return to her previous lifestyle. She is looking forward to preparing her next library exhibition, which will be on Mozart.

Rena has regained some movement in her left shoulder (0 to 90 degrees flexion, no active extension or adduction, 0 to 10 degrees abduction, no internal or external rotation), elbow (0 to 90 degrees flexion, no active extension), and hand (20 degrees wrist flexion; no active wrist extension, ulnar deviation, or radial deviation; approximately 10 to 40 degrees of flexion in all finger joints; no active finger extension). Some resistance to passive range of motion occurs in Rena's left shoulder during external rotation. She is able to grasp large objects with a left cylindrical grasp but does not have the hand strength to carry an object. Her poor distal finger strength does not enable her to use any other functional prehension pattern. Rena is right dominant, and the strength of her right upper and lower extremity is "good," meaning that she has full range of motion against gravity but is unable to maintain this position against strong resistance (Hislop & Montgomery, 1995).

Rena's left lower-extremity strength enables her to achieve 90 degrees of hip flexion, 60 degrees of knee flexion, and no active dorsiflexion. Rena's left leg is edematous. Her somatosensory status has improved since initial evaluation, with some gross lower limb tactile and proprioceptive sense.

Rena tends to ignore her left side and frequently does not realize when her left arm is hanging over the side of her wheelchair. She is now able to sit unsupported for 10 to 20 seconds, transfers from prone to supine to long sit with minimal assistance (she performs more than 75% of the task herself), and transfers from sit to stand and bed to wheelchair with moderate assistance (she performs between 50% and 75% of the task herself) (Hamilton, Granger, Sherwin, Zielezny, & Tashman, 1987).

Rena's long-term memory appears to be at premorbid levels, but her short-term memory is mildly impaired. She does not yet recall the names of the attending practitioners or the last time her children came to visit. She does, however, remember most events that occurred over the past 10 minutes. Her visual acuity and field of vision are intact, but testing of visual perception indicates deficits in this area. During morning self-care tasks you have noticed difficulties that likely can be attributed to poor form constancy, figure–ground spatial relations, and visual closure. She has some difficulty adjusting the position of clothing garments. Rena wears incontinence garments but has not soiled them during the daytime in the past 2 days. She sequences simple or routine activities but has great difficulty with complex unstructured chores or activities. Her topographical orientation around the hospital is also poor. Rena is still able to read and write. ■

3. Estimate how much Rena's cerebrovascular accident might influence her current and future engagement in areas of occupation and participation in contexts using Table 13.1 to record your expectations. Use the qualifiers to rate activity limitations; this scale was derived from the *International Classification of Functioning, Disability and Health* (World Health Organization, 2001). (Part of the table has been completed to provide cues about Rena's potential). Knowledge gained from experience with clients who have similar impairments helps occupational therapy practitioners construct an image of a person's potential.

4. During your discussions with Rena, she identified several aspirations, including caring for her children, regaining independence in BADL, managing her home, returning to work, and maintaining her relationship with her boyfriend Benjamin. Select one of these aspirations and complete the Activity Demands and Client Factors sections of the Client Profile and Task Analysis Form for one of the tasks that is essential to engagement in the desired occupation. Is there a match or fit among Rena's performance capabilities, the activity demands of this task, and contextual factors? Explain and justify your impressions. Identify potential activity demands, performance limitations, and contextual barriers that might limit her engagement.

a. Define goals and objectives for Rena's rehabilitation. Write out one of her goals in this area and three corresponding short-term objectives (a sample format is provided in Appendix K). In practice you would establish and prioritize these goals and objectives in collaboration with Rena, her family, and other members of the rehabilitation team.

b. Identify and describe potential intervention strategies and assistive devices. Appendix G lists approaches to intervention you could consider.

Table 13.1. Ratings of Rena's current performance and long-term potential.

Task	Current Performance	Long-Term Potential
Basic Activities of Daily Living		
Bathing, showering		0
Dressing		
Eating, feeding		0
Functional mobility		
Personal hygiene and grooming		
Sexual activity		
Instrumental Activities of Daily Living		
Care of others and child rearing		0
Community mobility		
Meal preparation and cleanup		
Home establishment and management		1
Shopping		2
Work		
Job performance		
Leisure		
Leisure participation		
Social Participation		
Family and peer interaction		
Community interaction		

Note. Use the following qualifiers to rate Rena's limitations in performing the activity: 0 (no limitation), 1 (mild limitation), 2 (moderate limitation), 3 (severe limitation), 4 (complete limitation).

c. Design a 30-minute session with Rena to address one or more of her goals and objectives.

d. You have other clients on your caseload with goals and objectives similar to Rena's. How might you design a group session to enable these clients to work together to attain their common goals?

e. Identify agencies and social support systems in your city or state that could provide resources to assist Rena in attaining her goals. For example, is public transportation available in your city to assist persons who use a wheelchair with community mobility?

5. Almost 5 months have passed, and Rena is attending an outpatient rehabilitation program. She walks short distances with a rolling walker and uses a manual wheelchair for community mobility. She is independent in dressing and personal hygiene with the use of assistive devices and has learned to compensate for residual physical impairments. Intervention focuses on continuing to improve mobility, work performance, home management, and adaptation to her impairment and altered performance patterns. Engagement in these tasks requires improvements in the motor performance skills of strength, endurance, and left-hand fine-motor coordination and in the mental functions of calculation, sequencing, decision making, and short-term memory. Rena's left shoulder, elbow, and wrist have an active range of motion within 20 to 30 degrees of full range. Her two- and three-point pad grasp strength with the left hand is rated as good. Rena just announced that her boyfriend Benjamin has proposed marriage. The wedding will take place in 6 months. Rena is determined to manage all of the arrangements and make her own wedding dress. She wants to have a traditional ceremony with about 20 guests. Select and design a purposeful activity for Rena aimed at building her capacity to achieve her goals.

6. Although research suggests that employers are making greater efforts to accommodate workers with disabilities, there has been little corresponding increase in levels of employment among this population of potential workers. The employment rate for persons ages 16 to 64 years who had a limitation in their ability to work due to a chronic health condition or impairment was about 29 percent between 1990 and 1995 (Kaye, 1998). The Bureau of the Census estimated that 31.4 percent of persons with severe disabilities were employed in 1997, as were 50.3 percent of persons with any disability. In comparison, 84.4 percent of those with no disability were employed (McNeil, 2001). As an occupational therapy practitioner, how might you contribute to the development of a return-to-work program? Who might be on Rena's support team during the process of job reintegration? What accommodations may be necessary to redesign Rena's job? What accommodations are necessary to enable Rena to work toward participating in a full day of work?

Learning Resources

Adaptive Driving Alliance: www.adamobility.com
Canadian Wheelchair Sports Association: www.cwsa.ca
Disabled Sports USA: www.dsusa.org
National Ability Center: www.nac1985.org
Wheelchair Sports, USA: www.wsusa.org

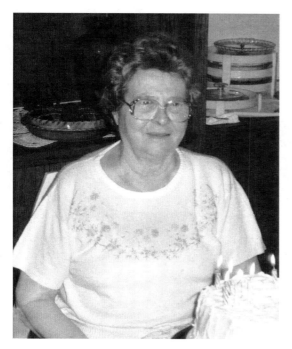

CHAPTER 14

Older Adults Living in the Community

Two days before my mother's 80th birthday I asked her how she wanted to spend the day. "I want to climb to the top of the Statue of Liberty," she replied. "Isn't there an elevator?" My mother looked at me. "I want to climb the stairs," she said.

—Remen, 1996, p. 173

CHAPTER OBJECTIVES
■ To show the use of logical thinking and creative analysis in developing intervention strategies to enable older adults to engage in occupations and participate in their customary contexts.
■ To describe how community resource agencies and social support systems can help older adults maintain their levels of engagement in occupation and participation in contexts.

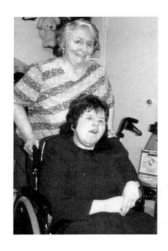

Older Adults Living in the Community

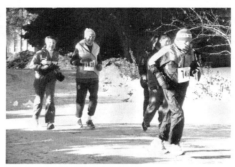

Life expectancy has increased dramatically over the past 100 years. Persons who are currently age 65 years can expect to live an average of 18 more years, and those age 75 years can expect to live an average of 11 more years (U.S. Department of Health and Human Services [DHHS], 2000). "This pattern, where each new generation lives longer than the previous one, is seen in many countries across the globe" (Jackson, Mandel, Zemke, & Clark, 2001, p. 5). Older adults now have fewer health problems and disabilities, live more independently, and live healthier lives than their predecessors (Chen & Millar, 2000; Menec, MacWilliam, Soodeen, & Mitchell, 2002). As life expectancy increases, health promotion and prevention initiatives focus on the need for older adults to maintain healthy levels of engagement in occupations.

People remain healthier for a larger portion of their life than previously, but because they will live longer, they are more likely to experience chronic disease or disability at some point during their lives (Fries, 1983; Jackson et al., 2001). The number of people ages 65 and older will increase from 35.6 million in 2003, or 12.6 percent of the population, to 53.7 million, or 16.5 percent of the population, in 2020 (Bureau of the Census,

2000). These increases in the number of older persons and in life expectancy, combined with the typical changes in client factors that accompany aging, have led to an increase in the prevalence of chronic disease and disability among the general population and activity limitations and participation restrictions among older adults (Figure 14.1). These demographic changes will continue, suggesting that the proportion and size of the population that has a disability will increase in coming years. By the late 1990s, almost half of older adults had a disability, and one third had a severe disability. The Census Bureau considered a person to have a disability if he or she had difficulty performing certain functions (e.g., sensory functions such as seeing, motor functions such as climbing stairs), activities of daily living (ADL), or certain social roles. A person was considered to have a severe disability if he or she was unable to perform one or more ADL, used an assistive device to get around, or needed assistance from another person to perform basic ADL (Bureau of the Census, 2000).

These demographic trends have given rise to the concept of successful aging as a key public health and policy concern (Fisher, 1995; Jackson et al., 2001). The characteristics of successful

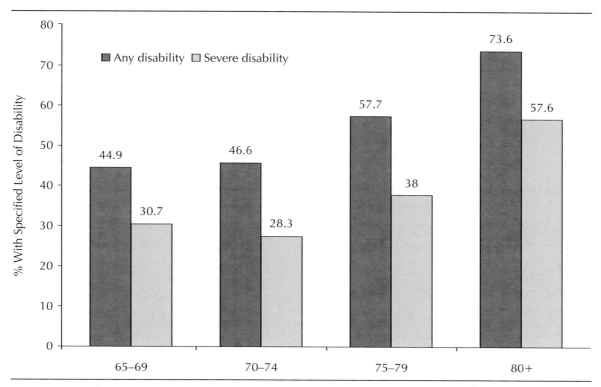

Figure 14.1. Disability prevalence by age, 1997.
Source: McNeil, 2001.

aging include low levels of disease and disability, high mental and physical functioning, and active engagement with life (Rowe & Kahn, 1998). Maintaining the health of older adults and the functional performance of adults with activity limitations and participation restrictions brings economic, social, and personal benefits to individuals, their families, and their communities (Bonder & Goodman, 1995; World Health Organization [WHO], 2001).

Role Transitions Among Older Adults

The roles and routines that people assume change across their life span, and each person's life story is unique. Typically, children become students when they enter school, adolescents become employees when they start their first job, adults become parents when they have their first child, and older adults become retirees when they leave the workforce. Engagement in occupations, participation in life situations, and role competency provide a sense of identity, add pleasure and enjoyment to

life, contribute to achievement, and help maintain the self and family life. Unfortunately, rapid changes in society may have left older adults without guidelines on the "proper way to age" (Jackson et al., 2001, p. 5).

Older adults may relinquish or experience a progressive loss of roles and occupations as they age. Many typical life changes place older adults at risk for social isolation. Retirement and losses of spouse and friends bring changes in roles and performance patterns that can affect the breadth and depth of social participation. Conversely, occupations that older adults celebrate and that produce a sense of self-worth often seem mundane to others (e.g., going to movies, reading). But these occupations are "salient occurrences in present life that often embodied meaningful themes" from the perspective of older adults (Zemke & Clark, 1996, p. 358). Individuals differ in the ways in which they respond to growing old, due in part to variability in personal experiences, societal expectations of appropriate roles, cohort effects, or personality factors that influence attitudes toward aging (Bonder, 1994).

Just as changes and transitions at other periods in the life span require persons to adapt, so too do the changes and transitions experienced in older adulthood. *Adaptation* refers to adjustments people make to enhance their ability to survive and thrive in the context of changing circumstances. Adaptation enables people to master life challenges and actualize their potential. It requires and is the result of changes in persons and their desired tasks and roles as well as personal and environmental contexts (American Occupational Therapy Association [AOTA], 1993; Mosey, 1986). Adaptation necessitates that people take an active role in responding to specific contextual demands and advocating for social change (King, 1978; Zemke & Clarke, 1996). Adaptation is also an occupational therapy outcome (AOTA, 2002).

People are living longer than ever before, and changes in society and everyday life are making past ideas about the process of aging obsolete (Jackson et al., 2001). However, the value people place on independence and autonomy remain tenacious in older adulthood. Although there are more older people, extended families are less able to provide informal care, in part because women are more likely to be in the workforce (Jackson et al., 2001). The challenge to society and communities, therefore, is to find ways to enable older adults to age successfully. Continued engagement in daily activities provides meaning and temporal rhythm in life (Zemke & Clark, 1996).

Occupational therapy practitioners, in collaboration with other professionals and service agencies, can address the health needs of the growing number of older adults who live in their communities through the design, implementation, and evaluation of cost-effective prevention and rehabilitation services (Anderson et al., 2000; Clark et al., 1997; Hay et al., 2002). Occupational therapy practitioners provide services to older adults who have or are at risk of having difficulty engaging in occupations and participating in contexts. They use task analysis as an evaluation and intervention tool to (a) identify performance patterns, performance skills, contextual variables, activity demands, and client factors that limit older clients' engagement and (b) target intervention strategies at barriers that limit and factors that support participation. Intervention approaches include health promotion, remediation or restoration, maintenance of performance capabilities, compensation and adaptation, and disability prevention (Appendix G). That older persons should be able to take part in the "naturally occurring activities of society" is a fundamental belief of the occupational therapy profession (AOTA, 1996, p. 855). After all, people of all ages place a priority on retaining independence and autonomy and having others witness and share their lives. Occupational therapy services directed at enhancing older adults' access to and engagement in occupations and participation in community contexts are consistent with this understanding of human motivation and behavior.

The Challenge

Read one or more of the case studies of Nelson, Paul and Minnie, and Gladys and Gene. Complete the questions accompanying each case. As you do so, consider the role of occupational therapy practitioners in promoting health and preventing disability when working with older adults.

1. You are an occupational therapy practitioner working for ABC Seniors Advisory Council in a community in which Nelson, Paul, Minnie, Gladys, and Gene live. The council's mandate is to maintain the health and independent lifestyles of older adults who live in the community. Assume that this community has the same supports for older adults as your own local community. How might you work with the council to enhance or enrich services and resources in your community that support achievement of the council's mandate? How might you work to ensure that older adults are linked with these resources? How might you design an injury prevention program in support of the council's goal to prevent falls among older adults in the community? If you would

like some assistance with this challenge, review the literature to identify the components of cost-effective injury prevention programs and review chapters 15 and 16.

How might you work with ABC Home Health, an organization that is likely to have a mandate similar to the council's? ABC Home Health has a tradition of directing services at individual clients, whereas ABC Seniors Advisory Council has a tradition of designing and implementing initiatives that enable older adults as a population to understand the qualities of occupations that contribute to health. If you would like some assistance with this challenge, review Clark et al. (1997); Hay et al. (2002); Jackson, Carlson, Mandel, Zemke, and Clark (1998); and Mandel, Jackson, Zemke, Nelson, and Clark (1999).

Health promotion and disability prevention can be used with individuals, organizations, and populations. Imagine that you work for ABC Home Health. What health promotion and disability prevention initiatives might you implement with Nelson, Paul and Minnie, or Gladys and Gene?

Nelson

1. Read the case study of Nelson and complete the Client Profile and Task Analysis Form provided in Appendix J. Occupational therapy practitioners are responsible for determining how impairment and activity limitation affect engagement in occupations and participation in contexts. These determinations or judgments are often based on limited information about clients. To develop knowledge and skills in this area, use the information provided in the case study and supplementary research evidence to predict the impact of Nelson's impairment and activity limitations on his engagement in occupations and participation in contexts.

2. Document specific, measurable, outcome-oriented client goals and objectives for Nelson (a sample format is provided in Appendix K). In practice, you would establish these goals and objectives in collaborative consultation with Nelson. Nelson has defined some priority occupations; predict whether they are achievable or not. Document your rationale. In what other meaningful occupations and roles might he have participation restrictions? Are these areas in which occupational therapy services might be appropriate to offer?

3. Identify a task in an area of occupation from the list of client goals and objectives and analyze the activity demands required for successful engagement and participation using the Client Profile and Task Analysis Form. First complete the Activity Demands section to analyze the task. Then complete the Activity Demands and Client Factors section and compare the information in the Level of Demand and Level of Impairment columns. Now, consider Nelson's customary environmental contexts. Is there a match or fit among Nelson's performance capabilities, the activity demands of this task, and contextual factors? Explain and justify your impressions. Last, identify potential activity demands, performance limitations, and contextual factors that might limit or support Nelson's engagement and participation in this customary occupation.

4. Develop an initial intervention plan to address the area of occupation you chose for Challenge 3. Select and design a purposeful activity or occupation-based activity for use with Nelson during a 30-minute session. Consider designing an intervention plan for the 2-week period prior to Nelson's discharge to prepare him for the demands that await him at home. Consider designing an intervention plan as if you were providing home health services after discharge.

5. There is an association among levels of physical activity, psychological wellness, and symptoms of depressed mood and anxiety (DHHS, 2000). Consider the following evidence and how it affects Nelson:

a. By age 75 years, 1 in 3 men and 1 in 2 women do not engage in regular physical activity. In fact, enhancing levels of physical

CASE STUDY: NELSON

Nelson is a 65-year-old widower whose wife died 3 years ago from a cardiac arrest. The couple did not have children, but Nelson is very fond of his nieces and nephews and their children. Nelson was a wheat farmer until he retired at age 60. He lives alone in his small farmhouse, which is about 10 miles from the closest town. He sold most of his land 5 years ago.

Nelson has had diabetes for 10 years. Over the past year he has had chronic skin breakdown on both feet. He recently underwent a left below-knee amputation and is now receiving occupational and physical therapy rehabilitation services at ABC Skilled Nursing Facility (ABC SNF). His medical history includes peripheral vascular disease, hypertension, cataracts, atherosclerosis, and peripheral neuropathy. Nelson's physician has suggested that he be discharged home within the next 2 weeks.

Before his wife's death, Nelson spent much of his day working on the farm and maintaining the yard while his wife managed the household and cooked all their meals. Since her death Nelson has assumed responsibility for all of these activities, but he was having increasing difficulty because of his inability to stand for long periods of time. During his leisure time, Nelson enjoys woodworking and riding his horse.

Although Nelson is walking with his temporary prosthesis in physical therapy, he mobilizes around the facility in a wheelchair that belongs to ABC SNF. Yesterday he walked 5 to 10 feet but relied very heavily on a standard walker because of poor standing balance. Both the physical and the occupational therapy practitioners feel that Nelson's problem with postural control is secondary to peripheral neuropathy in his right leg. His left leg is swollen, and his skin is slightly red after using the prosthesis for short periods. He has only limited interest in the rehabilitation program and speaks to staff during therapy sessions only after he is asked questions. During a conference in which Nelson's case is discussed, the dietitian indicated that Nelson appears to have a very poor understanding of an appropriate diet. Although he states that he cooks his meals, his answers to questions regarding his diet are vague. When Nelson is not in therapy, he spends most of his time sleeping or sitting alone in his room. He rarely converses with other residents at ABC SNF and has had few visitors.

The occupational therapy practitioner has been involved with Nelson since his admission, and services have been directed primarily toward achieving functional goals in basic ADL. Nelson is now independent in these areas using some equipment (e.g., bath chair). He performs these ADLs, however, from a wheelchair. The entrance to Nelson's home is not wheelchair accessible, nor is he interested in purchasing or renting "one of those clunkers."

Over the past week Nelson has commented that he has achieved all of his occupational goals. When instrumental ADL, work, and leisure interests are discussed, Nelson indicates that he plans to get to and from town by driving his truck, which has a standard transmission. "Once I am able to push the clutch down on my lawn mower and ride it, I can do the chores at home." Nelson indicates that there are several projects he would like to do after leaving ABC SNF, including painting the garage, tuning up the lawn mower, replacing the rain gutters, fixing the snowblower, and chopping wood for the winter. ■

activity has been defined as a national priority because of its protective effect on health (DHHS, 2000). Describe the role of occupational therapy practitioners in promoting physical activity among older adults. Does Nelson exhibit risk factors for reduced levels of physical activity? What health promotion intervention initiatives might you use with Nelson to address this area of health? What role might an occupational therapy practitioner take in designing intervention for a population of older adults to promote physical activity?

b. Six percent of older adults in America, or roughly 2 million of the 34 million adults in this age group, have a diagnosable depressive illness (National Institute of Mental Health [NIMH], 2001). Yet up to 15 percent of older adults who live in the community have depressive symptoms, and rates of depression in nursing homes are up to 25 percent in some areas. Depression is not an inevitable part of aging, but only 42 percent of depressed older adults seek help from a health professional (National Mental Health Association, 2002). Describe the role of occupational therapy practitioners in the prevention, detection, and treatment of depression among older adults. What are the risk factors for depressed mood or clinical depression? Does Nelson exhibit any of these risk factors? What health promotion and disease and disability prevention intervention initiatives might you use with Nelson to address the possibility that he is at risk for depression?

c. Major depression is the leading cause of more than two thirds of suicides each year (DHHS, 2000). Although the population of older adults was 13 percent in 1997, they accounted for 19 percent of suicides in that year. The highest rate of suicide, about six times the national average, is among White men age 85 years or older (NIMH, 2001). Describe the role of occupational therapy practitioners in the prevention of suicide among older adults, keeping in mind that depression is a risk factor for suicide. What are risk factors for dysthymic disorder or depression? Does Nelson exhibit any of these risk factors? What health promotion and disease and disability prevention intervention initiatives might you use with Nelson to address his high-level risk of suicide?

6. Opportunities for social participation may diminish with increasing age. Explore the social opportunities available and accessible to older adults in your community. What events and activities are offered? Are these events and activities accessible to people using wheelchairs for mobility? What health promotion and disease and disability prevention programs for older adults exist in your community? How might these options promote health and fitness?

Paul and Minnie

1. Read the case study of Paul and Minnie and complete the Client Profile and Task Analysis Form provided in Appendix J. Complete the Client Profile, Performance Patterns, Performance Skills, Contexts, and Client Factors sections of the form.

2. Occupational therapy practitioners are responsible for determining how impairment and activity limitation affect engagement in occupations and participation in contexts. These determinations or judgments are often based on limited information about clients. To develop knowledge and skills in this area, use the information provided in the case study and supplementary research evidence to predict the impact of Minnie's impairment and activity limitations on her engagement in customary and desired occupations and participation in life situations.

3. Document specific, measurable, outcome-oriented client goals and objectives for both Paul and Minnie (a sample format is provided in Appendix K). In practice, you would establish these goals and objectives in consultation with the couple. Minnie has described some areas of need in relation to caring for Paul; how does her impairment affect her engagement in occupations, participation in contexts, and role competency? How might occupational therapy services address the needs of Paul and Minnie as individuals versus as a couple?

4. Identify a task Minnie must perform to care for Paul and analyze the activity demands required for successful engagement using the Client Profile and Task Analysis Form. First, complete the Activity Demands section to analyze the task. Then, complete the Activity Demands and Client Factors section and compare the information in the Level of Demand and Level of Impairment columns. Now, consider Paul and Minnie's customary environmental contexts. Is there a match or fit among Minnie's performance capabilities, the activity demands of this occupation, and contextual factors?

CASE STUDY: PAUL AND MINNIE

Paul and Minnie have been married for 48 years and have four children and eight grandchildren. The couple are both in their mid-70s. Four days ago Minnie fell while gardening and fractured her humerus; her right arm is in a cast and will be in a sling for approximately 6 to 8 weeks. Minnie has great difficulty caring for her husband in this condition, and her family physician arranged for home health services. Paul was diagnosed with Parkinson's disease almost 20 years ago.

Minnie answers the door and introduces herself and her husband to an occupational therapy practitioner; Paul lifts his tremulous hand as if to wave hello from his seat at the dining room table. He is sitting in front of playing cards that are arranged in a row, face up and on the tabletop. The couple appear to have been playing a game. As the interview proceeds, Minnie contributes to most of the conversation while her husband watches. Minnie has a list of services and equipment that she wants, including an assistant to come and bathe Paul twice a week, someone to assist with housework, and a grab bar next to the toilet. Once provided with this assistance and equipment, Minnie expects that she will once again be able to take care of her husband.

When asked about her concerns regarding bathing and access to the toilet, Minnie indicates that she is unable to get her husband into the bathtub without the use of both arms. Although she assists him on and off the toilet, this task is very difficult for both Minnie and Paul, and since Minnie injured herself the task has become close to impossible. Paul has begun to wear incontinence pads, which is upsetting for him. The couple do not have any assistive devices for the toilet or the bathtub. Minnie indicates that Paul was given a walker 5 years ago, but in her opinion he walks better and is safer with her assistance because he is unstable with the walker.

Paul relies very heavily on his wife's assistance and support to get up and down from furniture and to walk. When the couple walk together from the dining room to the living room, the most difficult activity is getting up from the dining room chair. Minnie indicates "getting up is always the hardest.... After he gets going, we are pretty good together." Paul walks into the living room with a stooped posture and slow, shuffling gait; and his wife holds him close to her using her left arm. Once in the living room, the couple slows their pace before turning toward the piano. Paul sits on the piano bench and says in a quiet monotone, "It's easier to get up from here."

Minnie indicates that she is the "planner, organizer, and motivator of the family." "My husband and I spend every second Monday afternoon at the library. Paul does not read very much because he has trouble with the pages, but I love to read. On the way home we stop for dinner at a restaurant. On Tuesday or Wednesday we go out to the bank and the grocery store. My husband stays in the car while I do the running around.... Friday is our day for swimming, and my husband takes me out for an afternoon dinner date every Saturday. We often go to our favorite garden terrace restaurant. Sunday is our day of rest, although I am usually busy in the yard. By the end of the day we are usually ready to go out for a light dinner." Paul watches his wife as she describes their week together. Although he does not smile, he seems to be very interested in the conversation.

The couple live in a small, two-bedroom bungalow in the suburbs with two sets of stairs at the entrance of the home. The property has a very large lawn and a small garage. Before her fall Minnie drove the couple around in their small two-door car. They have gone out less recently, because they must now use a taxi to get around in their community. ■

Explain and justify your impressions. Last, identify potential activity demands, performance limitations, and contextual factors that might limit or support Paul in his engagement in occupations and activities Minnie no longer can support.

5. Develop an initial intervention plan to address participation restrictions in the task you have just analyzed. Consider the different approaches and types of interventions as well as outcomes applicable to occupational therapy practice (Appendixes G, H, and I).

6. Develop an initial intervention plan to address the couples' performance limitations. How might your strategies incorporate their individual and interdependent needs and priorities?

7. Explore transportation options for older adults in your community. Are they affordable to older adults? Do any agencies provide social participation opportunities to older adults who are mobile in the community? How about those who are confined to their homes? Are these activities affordable to older adults? Consider that the median income for older persons in 2000 was $19,168 for men and $10,899 for women, and 3.4 million older persons, or 10.2 percent, were below the poverty level in 2000 (Administration on Aging, 2001).

Gladys and Gene

1. Read the case study of Gladys and Gene and complete a Client Profile and Task Analysis Form (Appendix J) for both people. Complete the Client Profile, Performance Patterns, Performance Skills, Client Factors, and Contexts sections of the form.

2. Occupational therapy practitioners are responsible for determining how impairment and activity limitation affect engagement in occupations and participation in contexts. These determinations or judgments are often based on limited information about clients. To develop knowledge and skills in this area, use the information provided in the case study and supplementary research evidence to predict the impact of Gene's newly diagnosed impairment and activity limitations on his engagement in customary and desired occupations and participation in contexts.

3. Using the completed Client Profile and Task Analysis Forms for Gladys and Gene, determine the areas of need that should be addressed to ensure that both have their respective needs met. What is Gladys's potential to modify her occupational engagement and participation in contexts? What is Gene's potential?

4. Occupational therapy practitioners working in home health services are entering private homes and have the opportunity to observe family relationship patterns firsthand. Given the fact that Gladys expects to answer the practitioner's interview questions while Gene makes lunch, role-play how you might engage both partners in the interview and goal-setting process.

5. Document specific, measurable, outcome-oriented client goals and objectives for Gladys and Gene (see Appendix K). In practice, you would establish these goals and objectives in consultation with the couple. How might the occupational therapy practitioner address this couple's needs?

6. Identify a task from the list of goals and objectives that is a priority to both Gladys and Gene and analyze the activity demands required for successful engagement using their Client Profile and Task Analysis Forms. First, complete the Activity Demands section to analyze the task. Then, complete the Activity Demands and Client Factors section and compare the information in the Level of Demand and Level of Impairment columns. Now, consider the couple's environmental and personal contexts. Is there a match or fit among this couple's performance capabilities, the activity demands of this occupation, and contextual factors? Explain and justify your impressions. Last, identify potential activity demands, performance limitations, and contextual factors that might limit or support their engagement as a couple in this customary occupation.

7. Develop an initial intervention plan to address this area of occupation. Consider the different approaches and types of interventions as well as outcomes applicable to occupational therapy practice (Appendixes G, H, and I).

8. What type of intervention could be or should be provided through a home health service agency? Review Appendix G for assistance with this challenge. If you receive a referral to see Gene, can you provide services directed

CASE STUDY: GLADYS AND GENE

Gene is a 68-year-old man who was recently hospitalized after suffering a mild heart attack. For many years he has been the primary caregiver for his wife Gladys, who is severely disabled with rheumatoid arthritis. The family has requested assistance from ABC Community Health Services because Gene is experiencing difficulties caring for Gladys. Their only daughter, who lives 3 hours away, is concerned that Gladys may need to be placed in a continuing care center.

Gladys and Gene's home is a split-level design with the kitchen, dining room, den, and half bathroom on the main level and the bedrooms and a full bath on the upper level. There are two exterior stairs and six stairs between the main and upper level. As the occupational therapy practitioner enters the home to begin the evaluation session, Gene asks his wife what he should make for lunch. Gladys sits in an overstuffed antique chair that is positioned next to a window. From that position she can see the front entrance to the house, the garden, and the kitchen. Magazines, two candy dishes, a radio, and a television surround the chair. The practitioner observed Gene walk over to the candy dish, put two small peppermints in his wife's mouth, and leave the room to prepare lunch as directed.

Gladys has limited extension in all metacarpophalangeal (MP) joints and ulnar drift bilaterally. Although she holds her left MP and proximal interphalangeal joints in flexion, she has enough active extension in these fingers to hold an object 1 in. in diameter with a cylindrical grip. She does not wear resting splints at night because "they are too clumsy and look awful." Although she has a walker and reacher, they are of minimal use to her because of her inability to hold onto the walker and the amount of finger flexion and extension and strength required to grasp and squeeze the trigger of the reacher. Gladys walks very slowly around the home. She ascends and descends stairs with moderate assistance from Gene (Gladys can perform between 50% and 75% of the task). She tends, however, to spend the vast majority of her day sitting in the chair by the window. Although she has a wheelchair, it is used exclusively for community outings. The only other assistive device in use is a raised toilet seat.

Since the heart attack, Gene tires more easily and finds that he has to rest after making meals or doing housework. Vacuuming is particularly tiring. He seems to have energy only for Gladys's personal care and meal preparation and cleanup. He has difficulty helping Gladys in and out of the tub daily. Gladys truly enjoys her bath; "I don't know what I would do without my daily bath. It eases the morning aches and pains." Gene knows that Gladys loves her morning bath, but he must sit down for a few minutes after helping her, and he feels he can't continue. Gene no longer has the time or energy to work in the garden, an activity he enjoyed in the past. Community outings are particularly tiring for him, and lifting the wheelchair in and out of the car trunk leaves him exhausted and weak. They have always been able to accommodate Gladys's disability to ensure that they continue to have a sex life, but nobody has talked to them about sexual health care since his heart attack. Both are concerned about the effect the heart attack is having on their intimacy.

In the past, Gene and Gladys led an active life of gardening, hiking, traveling, and socializing with friends. More recently, Gene has continued to work in the garden for very short periods while Gladys sits and watches. They like to plan the annual garden during the winter months. Until the heart attack, they socialized on a regular basis and hosted a bridge tournament at their home once a month. Gladys has watched while Gene and their guests play the game. They are aware of their daughter's concerns about their ability to continue living at home. They are adamantly opposed to any move, although they understand their daughter's concerns and recognize that changes may be necessary. ■

toward Gladys? Review research evidence on the effectiveness and cost-effectiveness of home health services (home care services) for older adults. What are the characteristics of effective and efficient services?

9. Determine current and temporal trends in levels of home health services nationally and in your community. Become familiar with the availability and accessibility of home health and institutional care options available in

your community. How affordable are these housing options to older adults? Consider that the median income for older persons in 2000 was $19,168 for men and $10,899 for women, and 3.4 million older people, or 10.2 percent, were below the poverty level in 2000 (Administration on Aging, 2001).

10. Imagine that Gladys and Gene live in your community. Identify available community resources that serve the needs of older adults like Gladys and Gene (e.g., voluntary, advocacy). Given the information provided in the case study and your understanding of the role of home health services and other available community resources, do you agree with the daughter that Gladys should be placed in a continuing care center? What is your rationale? ■

Learning Resources

Department of Health and Human Services, Administration on Aging: www.aoa.gov

National Family Caregiver Support Program: www.aoa.gov/carenetwork

National Institute of Arthritis and Musculoskeletal and Skin Diseases: www.niams.nih.gov

National Institute of Neurological Disorders and Stroke: www.ninds.nih.gov

National Institute on Aging: www.nia.nih.gov

Resource Directory for Older People: www.nia.nih.gov/resource

IV

Health of Communities and Populations

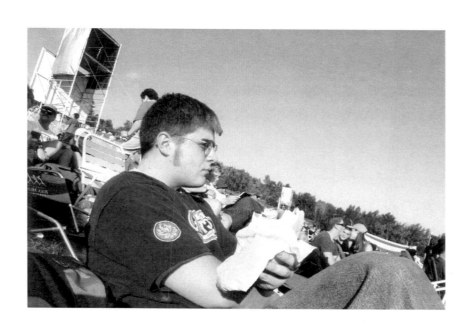

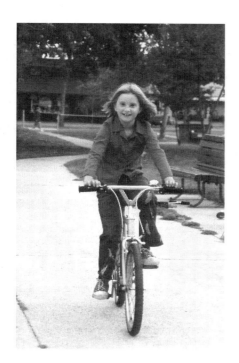

CHAPTER 15

Healthy People, Communities, and Populations

Achieving the vision of "Healthy People in Healthy Communities"... demands that all of us work together, using both traditional and innovative approaches, to help the American public achieve the 10-year targets defined by Healthy People 2010.

—Shalala, 2000

CHAPTER OBJECTIVES

▓ To define the similarities and differences among the medical, behavioral, and socioenvironmental models of health intervention.

▓ To describe the Healthy Communities movement.

▓ To outline the similarities and differences between the determinants of a population's health status and the foci of occupational therapy practice (persons, environments, and occupations).

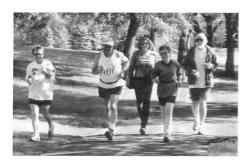

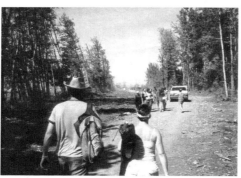

Healthy People, Communities, and Populations

Health professionals use several approaches to guide the development of interventions to improve health status. These approaches have evolved over time to include medical, behavioral, and socioenvironmental models of practice. People who use these approaches have made and continue to make an impact on the health of individuals and populations. When considering health interventions targeted toward populations, these approaches are indivisible, and all come into play.

Proponents of the medical model view *health* as the absence of disease, trauma, or other health condition and *disability* as an activity limitation or participation restriction resulting from a health condition or impairment. Health professionals who use this approach focus on individual clients and the management of physiological risk factors, disease, or impairment. Examples of interventions using the medical model approach to health maintenance would be to reduce activity levels to manage the risk of cardiac disease and to exercise to improve fitness and reduce physiological risk. Proponents of the behavioral model view health as being controlled by individuals; therefore, intervention focuses on promoting healthy lifestyles and addressing behavioral risk factors. Examples

of this approach to intervention include health education programs that teach clients about risk factors for cardiac conditions and ways to reshape their lifestyles to reduce their risk, or counseling programs that inform adolescents how to avoid tobacco and drug addiction and reduce their exposure. Public policies that require people to use seatbelts and bike helmets and public health monitoring to control the sequelae of schizophrenia are other examples of a behavioral approach to intervention.

Proponents of the socioenvironmental or ecological model view health as a function of social and environmental determinants. The premise is that changes at the community level, rather than the individual level, will have the most significant influence on the health of the population (Labonte, 1993; McBeth & Schweer, 2000). Health professionals who use this approach point to research and practice indicating that differences among populations in health status are attributable to variability in their exposure to ecological contexts that create and sustain inequities in health. Therefore, these practitioners direct health intervention toward altering socioenvironmental conditions to create healthy environments and improve health status.

Socioenvironmental models acknowledge that the health and well-being of a population go beyond traditional biomedical determinants of health to include broader conditions and resources for health in the social, political, cultural, and physical environments. Such conditions as peace, shelter, education, food, income, employment, literacy, a stable ecosystem, social justice, and equity are seen as key determinants of the health of populations (U.S. Department of Health and Human Services [DHHS], 1979, 2000; Wallerstein, 1992; World Health Organization [WHO], 1984, 1986, 2000). These determinants of health and wellness require health promotion strategies and a community development process. In comparison to biomedical and behavioral models, ecological models that rely on community-focused approaches to improving health change the focus from "us and them" to "us being them" (McKenzie & Smeltzer, 2001).

Community groups, associations, coalitions, and organizations are central to socioenvironmental health intervention models; communities implement their own health promotion and disability and disease prevention strategies. The socioenvironmental model views each community as a geopolitical entity with its own unique environment, personality, characteristics, power structure, health status, and resources for sustainable change (Kaufman, 1990; Labonte, 1993; McKenzie & Smeltzer, 2001). An example of a socioenvironmental intervention is a welfare-to-work initiative that covers an array of needs of dislocated workers through stress and financial management workshops, lessons on writing resumes and preparing for employment interviews, and employee assistance programs.

There are significant and necessary relations among medical, behavioral, and socioenvironmental models all necessary to address the complex phenomenon of health. After all, the goal of all three models of health intervention is to serve and fulfill society's interest in ensuring conditions to support healthy people, communities, and populations (DHHS, 1998; Kaufman, 1990; Labonte, 1993; WHO, 1980, 2001).

A Systematic Approach to Improving the Health of Populations

In response to international recognition that the health of North Americans and Europeans was not improving despite large and increasing investments in health care that focused on biomedical and behavioral interventions, the Healthy Communities movement emerged. Similarly, the Healthy Cities movement emerged from the WHO (1986) publication *Ottawa Charter for Health Promotion*. The Healthy Communities and Healthy Cities movements built their interventions on a merging of the medical, behavioral, and socioenvironmental models of health intervention, and these movements' philosophies have coalesced to become what is now the strategy for health promotion espoused by most health leaders, including the U.S. Department of Health and Human Services. The Healthy Communities movement seeks to build and strengthen multisectoral partnerships to improve the social and health conditions in the spaces where people live, advocate for the formulation of healthy public policy, maintain healthy environments, and promote healthy lifestyles (Pan American Health Organization, 2002). It "embodies healthy schools, workplaces, health care facilities, markets, and other settings.... It is a practical example of the effectiveness of partnerships between local governments involving different departments, residents, non-government organizations, private sectors, community organizations, and academics" (WHO, 1998, p. 20).

In 2000, DHHS presented *Healthy People 2010*, which sets forth 10-year goals and objectives that address the health of the nation. This document includes a conceptual framework entitled the Healthy People in Healthy Communities (HPHC) that identifies the DHHS's view of the determinants of health. As illustrated in Figure 15.1, these determinants include characteristics of individuals (e.g., biology, behavior) and their contexts (e.g., physical and social environment, policies and interventions, access to quality health care).

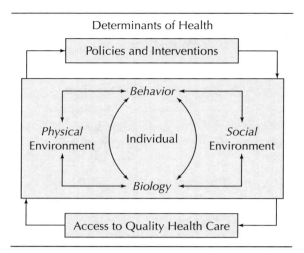

Figure 15.1. Healthy People in Healthy Communities Framework.

From *Healthy People 2010: Understanding and improving health* (p. 18), by U.S. Department of Health and Human Services, 2000, Washington, DC: Author.

The determinants of the health of populations defined in the HPHC Framework are strikingly similar to the dimensions of concern to occupational therapy practitioners as defined by the American Occupational Therapy Association (AOTA). Therefore, the domains and dimensions of concern to occupational therapy practitioners, as defined in the *Occupational Therapy Practice Framework* (AOTA, 2002), have been superimposed on the HPHC Framework (Figure 15.2). This figure clearly demonstrates the degree to which the determinants of a population's state of health are encompassed and congruent with the domain of occupational therapy practice. Occupational therapy practitioners strive to establish and optimize the fit among persons, environments, and occupations, and the HPHC Framework identifies factors related to the individual (biology, behavior) and the social, physical, and cultural contexts that must be optimized to promote and maintain health. As a result, the Healthy Populations Engaging in Occupations and Participating in Contexts Framework (HPEO) illustrated in Figure 15.2 provides a useful frame of reference that can guide the occupational therapy process for client populations.

In essence, the determinants of health of populations specified by DHHS parallel almost exactly the occupational therapy domain and dimensions of interest as identified by leaders of the profession. Occupational therapy practitioners who seek to influence the health and behaviors of populations can incorporate the goals, objectives, and intervention processes recommended by DHHS to help guide and focus their services on improving the health of

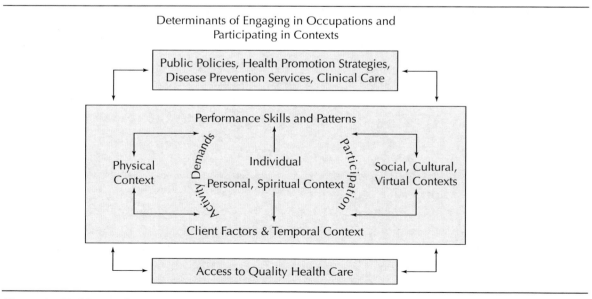

Figure 15.2. Healthy Populations Engaging in Occupations and Participating in Contexts Framework.

local communities to contribute to the improved health of the nation.

Health of People, Communities, and Populations: An Occupational Therapy Framework for Action

The primary focus of *Healthy People 2010* is on wellness. The goals and objectives articulated in *Healthy People 2010* focus on improving functioning, preventing disability, and enabling satisfying relationships as well as supporting a vital, creative, and productive citizenry (DHHS, 2000). *Healthy People 2010* articulates two goals: (a) to increase the quality and years of healthy life of the American population and (b) to eliminate health disparities among different segments of the population based on gender, race or ethnicity, education, income, disability status, rural residence, or sexual orientation. The focus, goals, and objectives of this national strategy for health parallel the vision and mission of occupational therapy. The primary focus of occupational therapy is on wellness "as a dynamic way of life that involves actions, values, and attitudes that support and improve both health and quality of life" (AOTA, 2001, p. 656). The profession is dedicated to enabling clients to enhance functional status, engage in occupations, participate in life situations, prevent disability, and promote health. The DHHS goal of reducing inequities in health parallels occupational therapy's consistent focus on providing services to vulnerable populations and persons most in need of amelioration of activity limitations and participation restrictions.

In addition to defining goals and accompanying objectives, *Healthy People 2010* includes indicators to help health professionals and communities target actions to improve health and to focus state governments, local communities, health care organizations, professional organizations, and others in targeting health care services, risk prevention programs, and health promotion initiatives (DHHS, 2000). The *Healthy People 2010* initiative has generated much interest in the concepts of health promotion and disease and disability pre-

vention and in activities and interventions that support attainment of its goals and objectives: "Imagine an integrated, holistic health system that serves people throughout their life span. Imagine achieving not just the vision but the reality of healthy people living in healthy communities" (McBeth & Schweer, 2000, p. ix).

Health services professions and organizations across the country and around the world are increasingly shifting from a focus on ill patients and disabled persons to a focus on keeping communities and populations healthy (e.g., American Medical Association & DHHS, 2002; WHO, 2000). Consequently, many professionals and organizations are designing and evaluating health interventions, and the materials they generate can be used in designing programs to achieve the vision of *Healthy People 2010*. For example, a *Healthy People 2010 Toolkit* is available to "provide guidance, technical tools, and resources" (Public Health Foundation, 2002, p. I). A *Community Planning Guide* is also available to assist community leaders in making their communities healthier and happier places (DHHS, 2001).

In keeping with this trend, the occupational therapy profession is evolving and undergoing a paradigm shift from an almost exclusive focus on clients as individuals to a more inclusive focus on clients as communities and as populations. Occupational therapy practitioners have always recognized the need to collaborate with clients, whether individuals or populations, to foster the development of performance skills and patterns required for engagement in occupations and participation in contexts. The transition of the occupational therapy profession toward a focus on communities and populations is emancipating and will ensure that the profession partners with communities and other disciplines to continue to make valued contributions to the health of the nation.

The Challenge

1. Familiarize yourself with *Healthy People 2010*. The Web address for this and other documents cited in this chapter are listed in the Learning Resources section.

2. Review two health intervention guides recommended by the DHHS, *Healthy People 2010 Toolkit* (Public Health Foundation, 2002) and the *Community Planning Guide* (DHHS, 2001). The National Library of Medicine, in partnership with the Public Health Foundation, developed a central Web site to make information and evidence-based strategies related to *Healthy People 2010* objectives easier to find; spend some time exploring this site.

3. Define the similarities and differences among the medical, behavioral, and socioenvironmental models and the approaches to health intervention they espouse.

4. Define the Healthy Communities movement and the interconnections of the medical, behavioral, and socioenvironmental models of health intervention.

5. What are the similarities and differences between the determinants of health of populations identified in *Healthy People 2010* and dimensions of the domain of occupational therapy practice?

6. Review the Occupational Therapy Services Model discussed in chapter 1. Describe how the intervention activities; targeted end of services; and immediate, intermediate, and ultimate outcomes of occupational therapy services parallel (or do not parallel) the medical, behavioral, and socioenvironmental models of health intervention and the Healthy Communities movement.

7. Consider the leading health indicators listed in *Healthy People 2010* (e.g., physical activity, overweight and obesity, mental health). Describe the implications these health indicators have for the practice of occupational therapy and the potential contribution of occupational therapy services to improving the health of the population in these areas of concern.

8. Consider the 28 focus areas identified in *Healthy People 2010*. In what areas might occupational therapy practitioners have a high degree of expertise? How might occupational therapy practitioners help to achieve the goals outlined in *Healthy People 2010* in at least one focus area?

9. Review the case study of Scott, the occupational therapy practitioner, in chapter 5. Describe how his work reflects the merging of medical, behavioral, and socioenvironmental models. Do you have any suggestions for ways the profession might increase its impact in Scott's area of practice?

10. Explore the work of the World Federation of Occupational Therapy, and identify its current initiatives in world health. ■

Learning Resources

Healthy Cities: www.hospitalconnect.com/healthy communties/index.html

Healthy Communities: www.nnh.org/HPHC/HPHC homepage.htm

Healthy People 2010: www.health.gov/healthypeople

Healthy People 2010 Community Planning Guide: www.health.gov/healthypeople/Publications/Healthy Communities2001/default.htm

Healthy People 2010 Toolkit: www.health.gov/healthy people/state/toolkit

Welfare-to-work initiatives: www.doleta.gov

World Federation of Occupational Therapy: www.wffot 2002.com

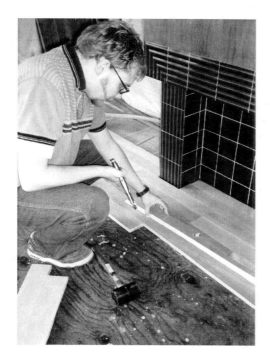

CHAPTER 16

Promoting Health and Preventing Disability

The health care system is offering occupational therapists a challenge to improve the health and function of the population. We can look at this challenge as a threat to our practice today, or we can see it as an opportunity to implement what the founders of occupational therapy envisioned—creating opportunities for people to lead independent and healthful lives.

—Baum, 1998, p. 43

CHAPTER OBJECTIVES

■ To define and distinguish disease and disability prevention, health education, and health promotion and to describe the emerging role of occupational therapy in using these approaches to intervention.

■ To describe how occupational therapy practitioners use task analysis in the context of health promotion and injury prevention initiatives targeted to populations.

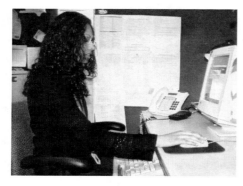

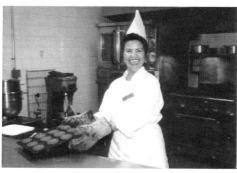

Promoting Health and
Preventing Disability

ealthy People 2010 established goals, objectives, and leading health indicators to help individuals and communities target actions to improve the health of the nation (U.S. Department of Health and Human Services [DHHS], 2000). The aim of this initiative was to focus state governments, local communities, health care organizations, professional organizations, and others on providing targeted health care services, health promotion strategies, and disease and disability prevention programs in areas of national priority. *Healthy People 2010* articulated two goals. The first goal, which addresses the changing demographics of the United States, is to increase the quantity and quality of life of persons of all ages. The second goal, which addresses the diversity of the population, is to eliminate disparities in health among segments of the population, which include "differences that occur by gender, race or ethnicity, education or income, disability, living in rural locations, or sexual orientation" (DHHS, 2000, p. 11). By undertaking this initiative, the DHHS sought to help people make informed decisions about their health and to foster the development of communitywide and statewide efforts to promote healthy behaviors, create healthy environments, and enhance access

to high-quality health care. "Given the fact that individual and community health are inseparable, it is critical that both the individual and the community do their parts" (DHHS, 2000, p. 10).

The nation's progress toward these goals is to be measured against 467 objectives in 28 focus areas. Ten leading health indicators that reflect major public health concerns were identified as the foci of the initiative: physical activity, overweight and obesity, tobacco use, substance abuse, responsible sexual behavior, mental health, environmental quality, immunization, access to health care, and injury and violence (DHHS, 2001). These health indicators represent major contributors to preventable causes of poor health and death. Measures of these health indicators constitute measures of the state of the health and well-being of the population; they identify major areas of concern for the nation and provide basic building blocks for initiatives designed to improve the health of the population.

The Contribution of Occupational Therapy

Injury Prevention

One of the DHHS's leading health indicators is injury and violence. More than 400 Americans die each day from injuries, and injury risks are so widespread that most people sustain a significant injury at some time in their lives. Although the causes of and risk factors for injury are broad, one of the principal contexts in which preventable injuries occur is the workplace. The Department of Labor's Bureau of Labor Statistics Census of Fatal Occupational Injuries estimated that 5.2 million workers were injured in 2001 alone (U.S. Department of Labor, 2002). The National Institute for Occupational Safety and Health (NIOSH) estimated that about 3.6 million occupational injuries were serious enough to be treated in hospital emergency rooms in 1998 (NIOSH, 2002). Additionally, NIOSH identified acute trauma as the leading cause of death and disability in the workplace. These statistics are astounding, and NIOSH intended their publication to motivate individuals into action and organizations into funding initiatives that reduce the incidence of injury and the disabling effects of injury-related impairments.

Health Education and Promotion

The growing emphasis on the health of populations over the past two decades has spurred an increase in health education, health promotion, and disability and disease prevention (Glanz, Lewis, & Rimer, 1997). These intervention strategies have been used to improve the health of individuals; local communities; and populations of people such as children, students, workers, older adults, and persons with disabilities.

Health education is aimed at closing the gap between what clients know promotes health (e.g., physical activity is good for one's health) and what they practice in terms of health behaviors (e.g., fitness habits and routines). Intervention is targeted toward promoting knowledge of healthy behaviors and contexts among individuals, organizational leaders, and policymakers. The intent is to facilitate healthy attitudes, behaviors, social structures, and contexts for living. Health education and awareness initiatives seek to "promote healthy behavior and lifestyle by increasing understanding of how

engagement in occupation can prevent illness and promote health and well-being" (Wilcock, 1998, p. 227). Health education has been described as a component of social action and health promotion that includes activities such as rallies, conferences, workshops, seminars, in-service training, health fairs, brochures, and circulars. These activities assume that "at least some people accessing the information will adjust behaviors as a result of the message" (Wilcock, 1998, p. 227).

Health promotion includes both health education and the provision of supports for environmental contexts that enable healthy behavior (Green & Kreuter, 1999). An empowering *health promotion* orientation holds that certain community processes are necessary to enhance personal health, and environments can be created that simultaneously protect health and support healthy personal behaviors (Labonte, 1993). Green and Kreuter (1999) suggested that health promotion is therefore "the combination of education and ecological supports for actions and conditions of living conducive to health" (p. 27).

The World Health Organization (WHO) (1986) described health promotion as the "process of enabling people to increase control over and to improve their health" (p. iii). It is "the science and art of helping people change their lifestyle to move toward a state of optimal health," and lifestyle change can be facilitated through intervention designed to simultaneously "enhance awareness, change behavior, and create environments that support good health practices" (p. iii). "Of the three, supportive environments will probably have the greatest impact on producing lasting change" (O'Donnell, 1989, p. 5).

This chapter provides readers the opportunity to examine the case study of Cam, an occupational therapy practitioner working in the community. This case illustrates the essential and significant difference between the provision of knowledge (i.e., health education) and the process of enabling people to improve their health (i.e., health promotion) in a participatory intervention process.

CASE STUDY: CAM

Cam, an occupational therapy practitioner, met on and off for a year with members of the board of directors of ABC Inner City Cooperative (ICC), a community organization that addresses the needs of homeless people who have substance abuse problems. During that time he collected research evidence that showed the magnitude of substance abuse among inner-city residents and the homeless urban population in particular. Armed with this information, Cam approached a subcommittee of City Council to legitimize the ICC's concerns, seek assistance, and request action. The subcommittee suggested several courses of action that seemed to Cam to be appropriate for ICC's board to consider adopting.

Cam convened a meeting with the ICC board members. After Cam presented the Council's recommendations and listed those he considered to be the most relevant, the board members quickly rejected them.

Surprised, Cam asked the board members why they rejected the suggestions. One person indicated that they lacked applicability. Another suggested that the overarching problem was that Cam and members of City Council had not included a broad sector of stakeholders in problem solving and in developing the recommendations.

Although many members of ICC's board of directors were less interested in working with Cam, a few remaining supporters asked him to continue to attend meetings as a guest. He worked with these supporters to gather a group of stakeholders that included inner-city residents, addiction counselors, local business leaders, a principal of the local high school, and the director of a local Planned Parenthood program. ICC's board members, in collaboration with these stakeholders, worked with Cam to develop a strong proposal for a health promotion campaign that included several initiatives. The ICC submitted

a budget for the campaign, and City Council accepted it for funding.

Cam helped the ICC design initiatives using information they collected through focus groups and participatory action research. They established the following services:

- a drop-in center for homeless adolescents that offered a warm environment, access to nutritious food from a local food bank, coaching in living skills, and addiction counseling;
- back-to-work programs that included assistance in seeking training, help with job searches, interest and aptitude screening, and résumé writing; and
- evening socials for young mothers that provided a venue for talking about the risks associated with exposing unborn children to alcohol and drugs.

After a few years City Council members and citizens applauded the success of this community-based health promotion campaign. ▪

Workplace Health

Adults spend a large percentage of their day at work, and workplaces are a prime location in which to influence health, including personal health. Many programs that encourage healthy behaviors are being designed and implemented at work sites, and the most effective workplace health programs are those that provide comprehensive programming and counseling (Heaney & Goetzel, 1997; Pelletier, 2001): "A comprehensive approach to workplace health involves the development of policies and programs that address issues related to the physical environment, the psychosocial environment, and individual health practices" (Bachmann, 2000, p. i). To implement a successful workplace intervention, organizations need to

- ensure that senior management supports and provides leadership on workplace health issues;
- designate various persons throughout the organization to be responsible for portions of the program;
- develop policies and programs that address the full array of issues, including physical and psychosocial well-being, work–life balance, and individual health practices; and

• recognize and influence external forces in the larger community that influence health (Bachmann, 2000).

Health promotion programs have been demonstrated to reduce employee-related health care expenditures and absenteeism (Aldana, 2001). Yet, although 44 percent of large work sites offer health promotion initiatives to their employees, only 25 percent of work sites with 15 to 99 employees offer such programs (Wilson, DeJoy, Jorgensen, & Crump, 1999).

This chapter provides readers an opportunity in the case study of ABC Doors-4-U to use task analysis and clinical reasoning to evaluate a work site and develop an injury prevention and health promotion program. After creating a profile of the activity demands and contexts of high-risk workers, readers can begin to define the factors that place this employee population at risk for injury. Readers can then plan intervention that incorporates the principles of injury prevention and health promotion, including health education.

It appears that low-intensity, short-duration educational programs aimed at increasing awareness of health and safety issues among employees may not be sufficient to provide desired change in improved health and reduced workplace injury. Yet there is strong evidence that individualized risk reduction for high-risk employees within the context of comprehensive programming and counseling is effective (Heaney & Goetzel, 1997; Pelletier, 2001).

Occupational Therapy Approaches to Health Promotion and Disability Prevention

Health promotion and disability prevention are occupational therapy approaches to intervention (American Occupational Therapy Association [AOTA], 2002), and the profession's adoption of these approaches parallels changing societal views about the importance of disease and disability prevention to the maintenance of health and wellness (Wilcock, 1998). AOTA "supports and promotes

involvement of occupational therapy practitioners in the development and provision of health promotion and disease/disability prevention programs. These health interventions and services may target individuals, groups, organizations, communities, and policy makers" (AOTA, 2001, p. 656).

Congruent with WHO policy statements, AOTA's (2001) position paper "Occupational Therapy in the Promotion of Health and the Prevention of Disease and Disability Statement" defined *health promotion programs and services* as a "planned combination of educational, political, regulatory, environmental and organizational supports for actions and conditions of living conducive to the health of people, groups, or communities" (p. 656). The *Occupational Therapy Practice Framework: Domain and Process* (AOTA, 2002) defined *health promotion* as an approach "designed to provide enriched contextual and activity experiences that will enhance performance for all persons in the natural contexts of their life" (p. 627).

By comparison, *disability prevention* is defined as "an intervention approach designed to address clients with or without disability who are at risk for occupational performance problems," and a *preventative approach* is "designed to prevent the occurrence or evolution of barriers to performance in context" (AOTA, 2002, p. 627). Primary health prevention programs and services focus on strategies, including health promotion activities, that are designed to help people avoid unhealthy conditions, diseases, or injuries. *Secondary prevention* includes early detection and treatment to prevent or disrupt the disabling process, whereas *tertiary prevention* is treatment and services designed to arrest the progression of a condition (AOTA, 2001). Many of the objectives outlined in *Healthy People 2010* seek to prevent activity limitations due to chronic health conditions. For example, one *Healthy People 2010* objective is to "prevent illness and disability related to arthritis and other rheumatic conditions, osteoporosis, and chronic back conditions" (DHHS, 2000, p. 55).

CASE STUDY: ABC DOORS-4-U

ABC Doors-4-U is a progressive firm that is dedicated to offering a comprehensive workplace health promotion program. The health promotion manager contracted Jared, an occupational therapist, to complete a risk analysis of the plant environment and to develop injury prevention and health promotion programs to promote back safety among employees. The firm's leaders were motivated to act following a recent workers' compensation board decision to increase the plant's insurance rates because of rising injury claims, over half of which were related to back injuries.

ABC Doors-4-U primarily manufactures wood doors but also provides installation services at large construction sites. Jared first interviewed the managers of the firm to determine the nature of past injuries. The health promotion manager described, among other initiatives, a program that ensured that all employees engaged in a health awareness activity for 5 minutes at the beginning of each day. The health promotion manager developed short fact sheets to promote discussion of health-related topics, and at the end of the discussion employees completed a form that asked how the presentation had affected them and what they could do to improve their health or increase their safety awareness. One company goal was to eventually have employees, rather than management, select the health promotion activities.

The occupational health and safety manager revealed to Jared that her primary concerns were the number of employees who exhibited a high degree of stress or symptoms of depression. Although the company has an excellent employee benefits program, use of these services is voluntary, and the manager cannot monitor the progress of employees who do engage the service.

Jared learned that the most prevalent claim was back injury due to repetitive lifting of weights over 50 lb. Jared then observed workers throughout the plant at different workstations to assess activity demands. At the first station, a conveyor belt moved large units of lumber to tables for cutting. Two men were required to guide 8-ft by 16-ft, 60-lb units of lumber as they were conveyed, then to lift them off the conveyor onto the 36-in.-high table. At the table one man sanded the lumber on one side using a power sander, then turned the board over to sand the other side. The same worker slid the lumber horizontally along the table to the next area, where the lumber was cut in two. Two workers were stationed to cut, one to guide the lumber into the saw and switch the saw on, and the other to guide the piece on the other side as it came through the saw. The next step was a fine sanding of each individual door, a one-man operation using power tools. Each door weighed approximately 30 lb, and one man carried each door to the staining booth.

Jared interviewed workers to identify their perceptions of risk. He noted as he talked to the workers that loud music interfered with his ability to hear their responses. Workers indicated that they were happy with their jobs, in part because they were encouraged to rotate through the stations to decrease repetitive action and mental and physical fatigue. They felt that their employer was generous in providing passes to the local fitness club to promote good physical health. They were given sufficient breaks throughout the day that allowed them to rest. a major concern they voiced was that it was easy to become lax in the work as it became more familiar, and that was when accidents happened. In addition, several workers had been in the job for over 15 years and were experiencing chronic back and wrist pain. The employer was eager for a prevention plan and was not hesitant about exploring options and costs. ■

The role of occupational therapy in offering prevention services to individuals and populations is linked to the profession's focus on the impact of the interaction among people, environments, and occupations on engagement in occupations and participation in contexts. AOTA (2001) articulated the following roles for occupational therapy practitioners offering primary prevention services:

• Evaluate occupational capabilities, values, and performance

- Provide skills development training in the context of everyday occupations
- Reduce risk factors and symptoms through promotion of engagement in occupation
- Provide self-management training in prevention
- Provide education regarding occupational role performance and balance
- Modify environments for healthy and safe occupational performance by promoting ergonomic workstations, exercise facilities for employees, safety policies, and the monitoring of employee work methods and practices
- Consult with industrial managers regarding the benefits of rest breaks, stress management, ergonomically designed work spaces, regular stretching, and proper body mechanics for factory workers
- Consult with businesses to promote emotional well-being by identifying problems with and solutions for balance among employees' work, leisure, and family lives.

The Challenge

1. Read the case study of ABC Doors-4-U. How can an occupational therapy practitioner's knowledge and task analysis skills be used to profile the unique characteristics of individuals among a population of workers at risk for injury, the activity demands of the job tasks, and the performance context of this industry? What dimensions of workers, their job tasks, and the performance contexts are of concern? Consider using the Healthy Populations Engaging in Occupations and Participating in Contexts Framework introduced in chapter 15 to assist you with this challenge.

2. Determine the incidence of workplace injuries and prevalence of work-related lower back disorders. *Incidence* refers to the proportion of a group initially free of disease, condition, or injury who develop the disease, condition, or injury during a specific period of time. Incidence is measured by identifying a group, examining the group over time to count new cases, and calculating the number of new cases relative to the size of the group. Incidence measures are typically reported for populations of 1,000 or 100,000 for 1 year. *Prevalence* refers to the proportion of a group who are experiencing a disease, condition, or injury at a specific time. Use information from the literature to identify factors that contribute to risk of injury. Consider starting your search at the Centers for Disease Control and Prevention's National Institute for Occupational Safety and Health Web site.

3. Review the "Occupational Therapy in the Promotion of Health and the Prevention of Disease and Disability Statement" (AOTA, 2001).

4. The client in the case study of ABC Doors-4-U is the population of factory workers who work there. To begin the evaluation, design an interview and develop an occupational profile to better understand the occupational history of the work site and the industry. What performance skills and patterns are required of the workers? Identify body structures and functions that are at risk for injury. Then analyze the activity demands of the job tasks and features of the performance contexts that promote or hinder engagement in occupations and participation in contexts at this work site. Consider using the Healthy Populations Engaging in Occupations and Participating in Contexts Framework introduced in chapter 15 to assist you with this challenge.

   To complete your analysis, answer the following questions:

   a. What are the physical demands of the job? What body structures and functions are required of workers while on the job? How might the physical environment (i.e., work site space) and objects affect performance?

   b. What process and motor performance skills are required for the job? Consider the concepts and objects used on the job, required actions, and sequencing and timing of the work.

c. What are the communication and interaction performance skills required for the job? What are the social interaction demands of the job?

d. What are the required performance patterns of the job? How might you determine whether there is a match between a person and an activity?

e. Identify the risk factors for injury within the context of the factory environment.

5. Define the long-term goal and measurable short-term objectives of an injury prevention and health promotion program. Consider that intervention can be targeted to workers, performance contexts, and job demands. In practice, you would establish the goals and objectives of a prevention program and develop the intervention plan in collaboration with stakeholders, who would both define priorities and identify opportunities for targeted intervention.

6. Consider the features of an injury prevention program to ameliorate the risks you identified in your analysis. What might be the features of a comprehensive workplace health promotion program for this workplace? O'Donnell (2000) suggested a three-step process for designing these programs: (a) prepare for the design process; (b) collect the appropriate data to plan the program; and (c) select the program content, develop the administrative structure, and outline the evaluation plan. Health promotion programs should address all domains of health and should include awareness, behavior change, and supportive environments. Sustainable programs are linked to business goals, supported by top management, and developed with strong budg-

ets. They include incentive programs, occur in supportive environments, and are rigorously evaluated. Finally, effective results are communicated broadly (O'Donnell, 2000).

7. If health education is a component of your plan, what educational modalities might work with this population in the context of the work environment?

8. What resources are needed to support implementation of the intervention plan and evaluation of its effectiveness? Identify policies that may support or hinder the implementation of the program.

9. How might organizational and industry leaders contribute to the achievement of broader health objectives among their populations of workers so that the industry contributes to the goals and objectives of *Healthy People 2010*? What might an occupational therapy practitioner do to provoke the interest and energy of these leaders? ■

Learning Resources

American Journal of Health Promotion: www.health promotionjournal.com

Centers for Disease Control and Prevention: National Institute for Occupational Safety and Health: www.cdc.gov/niosh/homepage.html

Health Promotion Advocates: www.healthpromotion advocates.org

Injury Maps at National Center for Injury Prevention and Control: www.cdc.gov/ncipc/osp/data.htm

National Center for Health Statistics: www.cdc. gov/nchs

National Center for Injury Prevention and Control: www.cdc.gov/ncipc

Web-based Injury Statistics Query and Reporting System at the National Center for Injury Prevention and Control: www.cdc.gov/ncipc/wisqars

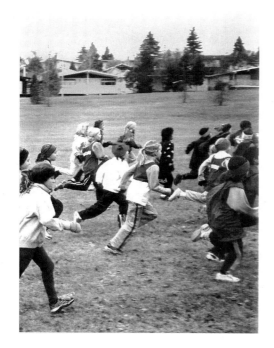

CHAPTER 17

Healthy Communities Through Community Development

*By locating our programs in the community defined
by locale or spirit, we are accepting the challenge of responding
to that community's need with what must be new
and innovative ways of being.*

—Fazio, 2001, p. 5

CHAPTER OBJECTIVES
- To describe how health promotion initiatives can be advanced through a community development process.
- To describe how occupational therapy practitioners use task analysis in the context of health promotion and community development.

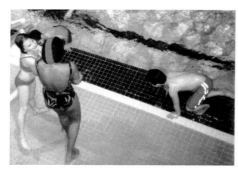

Healthy Communities Through Community Development

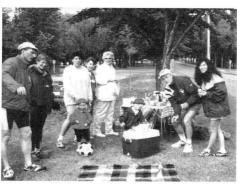

ealth promotion is the "process of enabling people to increase control over and to improve their health" (World Health Organization [WHO], 1986, p. iii). It is "the science and art of helping people change their lifestyle to move toward a state of optimal health" (p. iii). Lifestyle change is facilitated through intervention designed to simultaneously "enhance awareness, change behavior, and create environments that support good health practices" (O'Donnell, 1989, p. 5), and "new lifestyles are innovations that diffuse through the natural networks in a community by communication, and gradually lead to social change" (Puska, Tuomilehto, Nissinen, & Vartiainen, 1995, p. 40). Communities are not just geographic entities; any social aggregation constitutes a community, whether it be of students, persons with disabilities, older adults, or other persons with common interests.

Health Promotion and Community Development

The U.S. Department of Health and Human Services (DHHS, 2000) has observed and research evidence supports the idea that "over the years it has become clear that individual health is closely linked to community health—the health of the community and environment in which individuals live, work, and play" (p. 3). Therefore, health promotion initiatives increasingly focus on communitywide efforts to promote healthy behaviors, create healthy environments, and enhance access to high-quality health care. Raeburn and Rootman (1998) indicated that, to build healthy communities, the control of resources needs to be primarily in the hands of the people themselves. One example of a successful community development process that is recognized internationally is the North Karelia Project in Finland. Puska et al. (1995) summarized the process required to ensure positive outcomes related to lifestyle change in this community: "The gaping contrast between existing medical knowledge and the situation in everyday society stems from a host of formidable obstacles to healthy change—cultural, political, economic, psychological, and so on. The aim of a community program is to build a bridge for people and communities to overcome these obstacles, or at least to minimize them" (p. 32).

The development of good public policy and health promotion initiatives requires the juxtaposition of health professionals and coalitions working with communities to identify needs and priorities, establish a political voice, and work toward sustainable change with policymakers and organizational leaders incorporating the community will and research evidence into their decision making. The challenge is to link actions and create synergies among these stakeholders with the aim of building their capacity to empower the community to identify, lead, and manage strategies in support of health using available professional, institutional, and government resources. Head Start, Smart Start, and California's Children and Families Commission are exemplary initiatives designed to promote health and healthy life trajectories of young children through partnerships and joint initiatives among governments, organizations, businesses, and community leaders.

The establishment of a participatory culture among communities, health professionals, and policymakers requires a paradigm shift from a top-down consultation approach to a community-centered and community-driven approach. This cultural orientation is not unique to occupational therapy practitioners; health professions and organizations across the country and around the world are increasingly shifting from a focus on ill patients and disabled people to a focus on keeping communities and populations healthy (WHO, 2000). Occupational therapy practitioners who use health promotion approaches to improve the health of populations consider the "community" to be the client and use intervention strategies informed by the Healthy Communities movement (see chapter 15). The underlying philosophy of the Healthy Communities movement, the approach to health promotion and community development recommended by both DHHS and WHO, emphasizes starting where people live and creating healthy places to live, work, and play. Indeed, these health intervention strategies are appropriate to use whether services are targeted toward disabled populations (i.e., a community of similar people) or to all persons who reside in a specific location (i.e., a geographically defined community).

With all types of occupational therapy clientele, "the entire process of service delivery begins with a collaborative relationship with the client" (American Occupational Therapy Association [AOTA], 2002, p. 615). Clients define the goals and objectives of intervention and provide the primary resources and structures for sustainable change: "Community partnerships, particularly when they reach out to nontraditional partners, can be among the most effective tools for improving health in communities" (DHHS, 2000, p. 4). The case study of Vianne, an occupational therapy practitioner, describes the task of merging the perspectives of a community and a government-funding body in developing an integrated approach to health promotion and community-driven services to support healthy children and families.

Mobilizing Community Action

Earls (2001) observed,

> There is a broad recognition within most sectors of society that the quality of civic engagement is of critical importance to community effort to improve the health and well-being of children. This is true for all communities and families, regardless of their levels of material wealth and educational achievement. (p. 693)

James Heckman (2000), a Nobel laureate in 2000, recognized the fundamental social and economic importance of the early years of life:

> The best evidence suggests that learning begets learning. Early investments in learning are effective.... We cannot afford to postpone investing in children when they become adults, nor can we wait until they reach school age—a time when it may be too late to intervene. (p. 39)

Recent reports from the World Bank (Young, 2002), the Organisation for Economic Co-operation and Development, (2001), and UNICEF (2001) recognized that societal changes have altered the contexts in which young children are living and that integrated programs to restructure performance contexts to promote early childhood development are critically important to ensure that young children enter school ready to learn.

CASE STUDY: VIANNE

A Native American rural reserve community faced the closure of a public health unit that had historically offered services. Vianne, an occupational therapy practitioner, became the project manager responsible for re-establishing rehabilitation services for community members and ensuring their consistency with community values, one of which was the integration of health promotion initiatives for this population. Vianne worked with the community and federal funders to collaborate and develop consensus on a service delivery model. She understood that the critical components in service planning were communication strategies and cultural sensitivity. It was essential to bring together the perspectives of the community and the funder through collaboration, demonstration, and discussion.

Vianne served as facilitator in the collaborative development of an interdisciplinary service model through a community development process that ensured communication among the stakeholders. She interviewed key spokespersons to get a sense of the community's needs and objectives for services. The funder expected to provide conventional individual and small group rehabilitation services, but community members requested that the funder respect their interest in being responsible for their own health care issues and allow them to design rehabilitation services that would meet the distinct health and cultural needs of their community. Clearly, there was a desire among the community members that all initiatives have a health promotion focus and all services be based on a holistic concept of health that included mental, physical, and spiritual well-being, in addition to education, economic opportunity, and social participation.

Mental health services and parenting initiatives to promote performance patterns and skills in parents and communication and interaction skills between parents and children were priority community concerns. In fact, the community described mental health intervention as specifically encompassing health promotion and community development issues. Vianne remained flexible and responsive to the changing and conflicting demands by designing services that would evolve through phases and demonstrating how integrated services would work.

Vianne identified a natural starting point that would lead to a model that complied with the funders' mandate and that answered one of the health promotion issues of the community. As a result of historic decisions to separate native youths from their communities for the purposes of education and cultural assimilation, a generation

This chapter provides readers an opportunity in the case study of Community Action Toward Children's Health (CATCH) to practice using task analysis and clinical reasoning to set goals and objectives with a community. Unlike the protagonists of other case studies in this book, CATCH is not hypothetical; it is an exemplary community development initiative designed to promote health among children. The CATCH Web site provides information on the progress and success of its community partnerships, and this chapter's challenges require readers to step back and participate in the beginning of a community development process undertaken by CATCH stakeholders and partners. A task analysis approach will be used to frame an occupational therapy practitioner's contribution.

Occupational therapy practitioners offer a unique approach to assessing community needs, assets, and resources by conducting task analysis of population characteristics (i.e., persons), environments (i.e., performance contexts), and community actions (i.e., tasks and activities) that support or hinder health. Just as the concept of person–environment–occupation (PEO) fit guides the establishment of a client profile and analysis of occupational performance for individual clients, this construct remains applicable to community clients. The creation of a client profile for communities is referred to as *asset mapping*. At the community level, the PEO model translates to a community–context–action model. The community is a collective of people with performance skills and patterns, and body structures and funcof the community's members grew up in boarding schools away from their parents. This generation had now become parents, and many had not had the opportunity to develop parenting skills through role modeling. An interdisciplinary team worked with the community to integrate a parenting program into all intervention sessions with children; children received the mandated services, and their parents received services to enhance their success in child rearing. Many of the mental health issues appeared to be related, at least in part, to the impact of the parents' early childhood experiences and the stresses of raising their own children without a foundation of exposure to parenting performance patterns.

The service outcome demonstrated that, through innovative approaches, the fixed amount of funding available for individuals could be spread across families. Community leaders had the evidence to support parenting programs, which were sanctioned and funded as a result of the evidence-based outcomes. The idea of parent education sessions so inspired two community spokespersons who worked in the education system that they too designed opportunities and materials for use with parents during school events involving parents. Another community representative who was a member of the Band Council and an employer of many parenting-age adults encouraged the community to establish a day care center to support working parents and to provide respite options for other parents.

The program was so successful that the Band Council sanctioned other initiatives that various members of the community took the lead in developing. The day care coordinator developed nutrition educational materials for the children and their parents in collaboration with a local nutritionist to respond to the growing prevalence of diabetes and obesity among all community members. She also initiated family picnic days and included the parents and children in the menu planning. One by one, community members began to identify and act on opportunities to contribute to the development of parenting skills among parents in the community and to nurture healthy families. By meeting regularly, the spokespersons began to identify the initiatives that were most effective in achieving the goals they had for improving the health of the community. Over time, the policymakers began to identify and support the mechanisms the community identified as effective interventions to improve health. ■

tions are analogous to the community's assets. The context includes cultural, physical, social, temporal, and virtual environments as well as personal factors such as values, beliefs, and goals. The targeted action or occupation of a community is its members' level of participation in healthy lifestyles and behaviors. The occupational therapy process with individual clients involves assessing and optimizing the interaction and fit among person, environment, and occupation, and this procedure is equally applicable with community clients.

The process of mobilizing key individuals to assess the community's needs, strengths, and resources is a necessary requisite to the establishment of intervention goals, objectives, and priorities, which in turn become the vision, goals, and guiding principles embedded in service delivery. The challenge of sustaining community involvement in the process of change is best met by agreeing as early as possible on a vision for the community. This vision should emerge from the most important needs, values, and goals identified by the community (DHHS, 2001). The evaluation and intervention process is always client directed in that services focus on the priorities identified by key stakeholders in the community: "When community coalitions work together to set priorities and to allocate resources to these priorities, they are far more likely to continue to participate in the process and to achieve measurable results" (DHHS, 2001, p. 12).

Many organizations and people are designing health interventions that can be used to achieve the vision of improving the health of the nation as articulated in *Healthy People 2010* (DHHS, 2000). For example, DHHS (2001) published a *Community Planning Guide* to assist community leaders "who embark on a significant journey to make our communities healthier and happier places" (p. i). A five-step process of community development called MAP-IT recommends the following:

1. *Mobilize* key persons who care about the health of the community.
2. *Assess* areas of greatest need in the community and strengths and resources that can be tapped to address these areas (i.e., asset mapping).
3. *Plan* your approach by starting with a vision and adding strategies and action steps.
4. *Implement* the action plan using concrete steps that can be monitored and will make a difference.
5. *Track* progress and outcomes over time. (DHHS, 2001).

The Challenge

1. Read the case study describing CATCH and review the Web site (www.catch.silk.net) for this community development initiative. Consider the five-step MAP-IT process (www.health.gov/healthypeople/publications/HealthyCommunities2001/default.htm) as it applies to CATCH.
2. Key persons who care about the health of the community and its children have been mobilized around the vision to assist children of young families to the best possible future (Step 1 in MAP-IT). Individuals and organizations must be mobilized to form a communitywide coalition that will serve as an advocate or proxy to identify the needs and priorities of the community and as a catalyst and vehicle for establishing sustainable change. It is easiest to mobilize potential coalition members around issues that are already of special interest to them and to the community. According to DHHS (2001), "Local organizations are valuable because of their influence, their re-

sources, their involvement in the community, and the respect they command. They can support needed actions and they can mobilize resources to help implement such actions" (p. 9). How might you help the community partners in the case study bring a "dream team" together? What social groups or organizations might be available to assist with the process in your community?

3. At one point persons involved in CATCH met to assess areas of need in the community and strengths that could be tapped to address areas of priority (Step 2 in MAP-IT). Asset mapping involves identifying these community structures, resources, and functions so that intervention strategies can be targeted to areas most likely to lead to the desired outcome. In the context of CATCH, this desired outcome is the best possible future for children and young families. Asset mapping is a team activity, and the first stage is to identify potential team members among the community's citizens, professionals, organizations, researchers, and policymakers. How could you use task analysis to help these partners better understand the community (i.e., persons), environments (i.e., performance contexts), and actions (i.e., occupations) that support or hinder the futures of children and young families? How might you "teach" a team the concept of task analysis and its utility?

   It may be important to share research evidence to show and support community leaders in identifying the issues that are of real and immediate importance (DHHS, 2001). Explore the literature to determine factors that threaten the healthy development of children and families in the United States (the National Institute of Child Health and Development Web site, www.nichd.nih.gov, is a good resource). What areas of health has the DHHS (2000) identified as important? Are these areas applicable to children and families in your community?

4. CATCH planned an approach by starting with a vision, goals, and objectives and adding

CASE STUDY: COMMUNITY ACTION TOWARD CHILDREN'S HEALTH (CATCH)[1]

Community Action Toward Children's Health emerged in 1999 as a network with the mission of "working together for the health development of all children in the early years" (CATCH, 2001, p. 7). As portrayed in their theme bus (see Figure 17.1), this community coalition acts on several themes at once. By June 2000, CATCH had more than 100 community organizations and government agencies working in collaboration. These partnerships and teams formed around common values and needs and a convergence in perspectives that child health and development determine future health and success in life.

The Central Okanagan community is located in the interior of the province of British Columbia, Canada, and has a population of 150,000, including a mix of urban and rural residents. It is located about 250 miles from a major metropolis. Because the area attracts professionals, the number of service providers is generally sufficient across disciplines; however, there is no specialized children's hospital in the area. Tourism and agriculture are the primary industries;

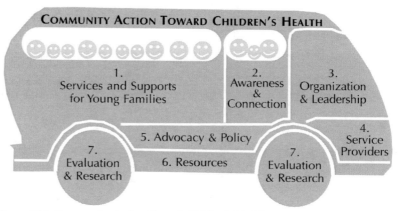

Figure 17.1. Community Action Toward Children's Health: Action themes.

therefore, the population size and characteristics vary seasonally with the ebb and flow of tourists, summer residents, and migrant farm workers. There is significant variability in socioeconomic status among families.

CATCH's collective vision is expressed in its charter and envisions a community in which

- all children are safe, secure, and loved and have the opportunity to develop to their fullest potentials free of limitations from preventable conditions;
- all parents are knowledgeable, motivated, and effective in their parenting role;
- all community members value children and parenting and take collective responsibility for child health and development; and
- all organizations and people share a common vision and work together effectively.

The goals of CATCH are to serve and support young families, create awareness and connection with the community, develop leadership within the community to ensure advocacy for children's health and the development of effective policy, involve service providers in the coalition, create and sustain community resources, and measure and monitor growth in community capacity. The mission was to develop the capacity for self-sustaining action within a 6-year period.

CATCH's founding members believed that the community had the assets it needed for success and that human resources were plentiful, including volunteer and paid service providers who were "skilled, compassionate, and eager to learn" (CATCH, 2001, p. 9). The challenge was to "find, build, release, and focus our assets effectively" (p. 9). ▪

---

[1]With permission from Dr. Eugene Krupa, CATCH Facilitator, and the CATCH Leadership Team.

strategies and action steps (Step 3 in MAP-IT). Use the information from the case study about the vision of CATCH to formulate client goals and objectives (see Appendix K) in support of attaining the community's vision. When work-ing with communities to establish visions, goals, and objectives, consider the following: Have all stakeholders contributed to the identification of the needs and the establishment of a vision? Is there consensus on the priority of needs? How might consensus be attained, and is it necessary? What outcomes are envisioned, and how might the outcomes benefit all sectors of the community?

5. Once goals and objectives were established, members of CATCH designed strategies and action steps in areas thought to have the most impact on attaining the vision (Step 3 in MAP-IT). How can task analysis be used to identify the dimensions of the community (i.e., persons), the environment (i.e., performance contexts), and collective actions (i.e., occupations) that hinder or support attainment of the vision? Are any of the occupational therapy approaches to intervention appropriate for use in promoting or supporting the development of healthy communities? How might occupational therapy practitioners use this information to assist the community in establishing an action plan?

6. Community partners are the vehicles through which strong leadership emerges, priorities and plans are established, and resources are mobilized in support of implementation. Implementation of the action plan should occur in concrete steps that can be monitored and will make a difference (Step 4 in MAP-IT). Leadership, action plans, and resources are required for sustainable change. Imagine that one of the community dimensions identified for intervention was the context in which children play. Now imagine that CATCH is located in your community. Define a goal for your community and objectives in support of this goal. What might be some concrete steps that members of CATCH could undertake in your community?

7. Communities should track progress and outcomes over time (Step 5 in MAP-IT), plan "early wins" to celebrate accomplishments, and share success stories. The process of creating a healthy community takes time, and the process of defining and redefining action plans is iterative as progress toward goals and objectives is monitored. There is no one way to provoke change, and many steps may need to be taken again and again. It is the community partners who will stimulate and sustain community action, development, and change. And it is through the process of tracking progress and monitoring outcomes that action plans remain focused on areas of continuing need and intervention plans result in desired outcomes. Given the goals, objectives, action plan, and concrete steps you defined for the community in Challenge 6, how would you track progress?

8. What do exemplary community development initiatives such as CATCH, Smart Start, and California's Children and Families Commission have in common? Describe the roles of occupational therapy practitioners in contributing to these initiatives to improve the health of populations. ■

Learning Resources

California's Children and Families Commission: http://ccfc.ca.gov

CATCH: www.catch.silk.net

Head Start: www.acf.dhhs.gov/programs/hsb

National Institute of Child Health and Development: www.nichd.nih.gov

OECD Report 2001. Starting Strong: Early Childhood Education and Care: www.childcare canada.org/policy/polstudies/int/OECDstrong.html

Smart Start: www.ncsmartstart.org

UNICEF Report 2001. State of the World's Children 2001: www.unicef.org/SOWC01

World Bank Report 2002. From Early Child Development to Human Development: www.worldbank.org/children.ECDtoHuman Development.pdf

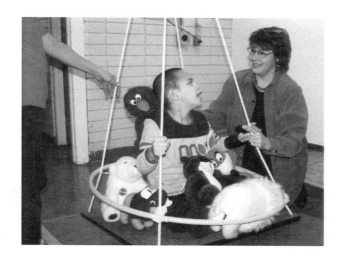

CHAPTER 18

Grounding Community Health Interventions in Evidence

Occupational therapists with a well-developed concept of the relationship between people's engagement in occupation and health are a primary source of expertise for research and developing public health practice based on the relationship.

—Wilcock, 1998, p. 221

CHAPTER OBJECTIVES

■ To describe how research evidence contributes to task analysis when services are directed toward client populations.

■ To describe how occupational therapy practitioners use research and relevant evidence in planning health interventions.

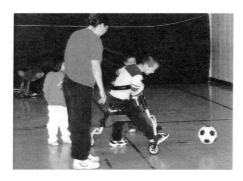

Grounding Community Health Interventions in Evidence

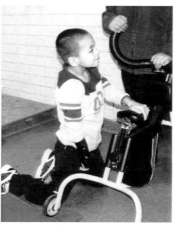

Intervention plans that are designed by occupational therapy practitioners to improve the health of individuals or populations must be built in collaboration with clients, designed to address targeted outcomes, and grounded in science. The challenge and rewards of evidence-based practice is in the process of accessing, evaluating, and using evidence to inform intervention plans and demonstrate positive outcomes for clients. To ground health interventions in science, practitioners must search out evidence relative to their practice and incorporate research findings using their own judgment and in consultation with clients (Law, 2002a).

In addition, practitioners can contribute to or conduct research to generate new practice knowledge. For instance, occupational therapy practitioners can use research-generated information to profile levels of engagement in occupations, to identify risk factors for poor health, to determine key factors to improve health, to provoke action to address key health issues, to establish baseline measures against which to track progress, and to assess the effectiveness of alternative intervention strategies. Evidence-based practice is a process that involves the merging of information, evidence, and judgment. It contributes to informed decision making and accountable intervention planning and implementation.

Accessing Evidence

Whereas information on individuals is obtained through interviews and assessments, information on communities comes through population-based research methods. Population-level information can be used to profile levels of health and wellness, performance skills, performance patterns, morbidity and mortality, performance contexts, and so forth. Research evidence can be used to identify factors that contribute to health, such as engagement in occupation, or conditions that put people at risk for ill health, such as reduced levels of physical activity. For example, population-based information can be used to determine the proportion of people who are independent in activities of daily living, who have work-related disabilities, who participate in sports, who participate in social events, and who are literate, as well as the prevalence (the proportion of a group who experience a disease, condition, or injury at a specific time) and incidence (the proportion of a group initially free of disease, condition, or injury who develop the disease, condition, or injury during a specific period) of health determinants such as disease, disability, obesity, substance abuse, unsafe sexual practices, smoking, and so forth.

Population-level statistics regarding health, performance skills, performance patterns, morbidity, and environmental contexts are typically reported for geographic jurisdictions or special populations (e.g., children, students, older adults). For example, the World Health Organization (WHO; www3.who.int/whosis/menu.cfm) publishes population-level statistics for countries, whereas U.S. federal departments such as the Bureau of the Census (www.census.gov) and the U.S. Department of Education, National Institute on Disability and Rehabilitation Research (www.ed. gov/offices/OSERS/NIDRR) provide population-level information for geographically defined or special populations such as persons with disabilities.

Population health research can be used to identify the origins and determinants of health, whereas epidemiological research seeks to identify the origins of disease, impairments, and disability. Both forms of scientific inquiry profile the prevalence, incidence, and temporal trends in health, illness, and other factors that contribute to different states of health and can be used to focus interventions on key issues and factors deemed to be significant determinants of activity limitations and participation restrictions. Program evaluation research can be used to track performance and achievement relative to the goals and objectives of services, as well as to identify effective health intervention strategies.

Using Evidence

Practitioners must combine the insights they derive from research with information on the performance patterns, activity demands, and unique contexts of a community gained through observation, focus groups, and conversations with community advocates. This combined evidence can then help the practitioner establish community needs, focus attention on the most significant issues, set priorities, target outcomes, and monitor progress. Just as the U.S. Department of Health and Human Services (DHHS, 2000) has set health goals and objectives for the nation on the basis of population health statistics, occupational therapy practitioners and their community partners should focus health intervention goals, objectives, and activities on the basis of the research evidence they gather.

Interesting research findings can be used to prompt a community into action. For example, health education strategies that focus on communicating the prevalence of substance abuse among pregnant women, the link between parental substance abuse and infant health, and the incidence of fetal alcohol syndrome can stimulate a community to action. This chapter provides readers the opportunity to consider an initiative undertaken in one such community in the case study of Rebecca, an occupational therapy practitioner.

Generating Evidence

Population health researchers seek to identify the origins and determinants of health. Occupational therapy practitioners have a role in contributing to this research by encouraging and supporting critical appraisal of their own hypotheses about the value of engagement in occupations and participation in contexts. One hypothesis, for example, is that the fit among persons and their environments and occupations contributes to health. Another hypothesis is that the performance of meaningful activities is key to health, functioning, and quality of life. Occupational therapy practitioners have led and participated in investigations that test these hypotheses (Clark et al., 1997; Hay et al., 2002; Jackson, Carlson, Mandel, Zemke, & Clark, 1998).

There is a growing understanding in the research community that some risk behaviors

CASE STUDY: REBECCA

Rebecca's occupational therapy practice was inner city and community based. Over time she noticed the high prevalence of fetal alcohol syndrome (FAS) in children and wondered if many of the young adults on her caseload had also had prenatal substance exposure. She did some research on the incidence and prevalence of FAS across the country and in her state and city in particular. The statistics were alarming. Maternal alcohol use during the prenatal period is one of the leading causes of preventable health conditions among children (Centers for Disease Control and Prevention, 2002). Estimates of the prevalence of FAS range from 0.3 to 2.2 cases per 1,000 births, and many more children are born with alcohol-related neurodevelopmental disorders. Maternal risk factors include being unmarried, a smoker, age 25 years or older, college educated, and a frequent binge drinker, as well as exposure to social contexts that involve drinking (Floyd, Decoufle, & Hungerford, 1999; May & Gossage, 2001).

Children exposed to alcohol during intrauterine development often have a wide range of impairments of body structures and functions and have lifelong developmental consequences such as mental retardation, learning disabilities, and serious behavioral problems. There is little consensus on these consequences, however, because substance-exposed infants are also influenced over their life courses by their environmental contexts and their alcohol and drug consumption patterns. Birth defects associated with prenatal alcohol exposure can occur in the first few weeks of pregnancy, before a woman knows she is pregnant. One study found that 45 percent of women consumed alcohol during the 3 months before they found out they were pregnant, and 1 in 20 drank at moderate to heavy levels (Floyd et al., 1999). Estimates of annual health care costs associated with FAS were $2.8 billion in 1998 (CDC, 2002). One of the national health objectives in *Healthy People 2010* is to reduce the incidence of FAS (objective no. 16–18; DHHS, 2000).

Rebecca had a strong working relationship with members of the community, who often asked her to present workshops on rehabilitation programs and intervention strategies. She took advantage of this option to develop a series of presentations and to challenge the community to develop a unique FAS prevention strategy that included health promotion principles and a community development process. She was aware that universal health education initiatives that had occurred during the 1990s had not decreased the incidence of FAS in her state, but she hypothesized that more comprehensive prevention initiatives targeted at high-risk groups might be effective and appropriate for her community.

Eventually the community adopted the challenge of reducing the incidence of FAS. It was clear to community leaders and to Rebecca that the prevention initiatives they knew about focused almost exclusively on information to girls and women. There was no social or educational initiative that included the men, and men were considered by the dominant ethnic group in their inner city to be protectors and providers. Therefore, initiatives were also designed to influence men and engage them in ways that would protect unborn children. Workshops for boys and men were established to provide opportunities to discuss their role in discouraging alcohol use by their partners before and during pregnancy and to practice safe sex, particularly when their partners had consumed alcohol or drugs. Community work programs for care of people with FAS employed men from the community. The role of these men was to link people with FAS to programs in the community, and they often helped transition former prisoners who had been diagnosed with FAS from correctional institutions to community programs. Bar vouchers with salient health education messages were furnished to men and women for use in obtaining free nonalcoholic beverages. All of the initiatives were funded as a Healthy Communities project.

Over time Rebecca assisted the community in developing an outcome evaluation process that had the potential to add to existing empirical and qualitative research on FAS. The community appreciated the opportunity to communicate, celebrate, and share their results with others. Evaluative efforts first focused on early wins and on communicating successes by monitoring changes in alcohol consumption patterns. ■

(e.g., substance abuse) are influenced by a combination of personal motives (i.e., personal context) and societal values, social organization, and culture (i.e., environmental contexts) (DHHS, 1998; Wilcock, 1998; Zemke & Clark, 1996). Occupational therapy practitioners have participated in investigations that link moral perspectives and occupational understanding to health; these investigations are of unique value to understanding factors that influence the health of populations (Fazio, 2001; Wilcock, 1998; Zemke & Clark, 1996).

To conduct research to test hypotheses regarding linkages among people and their occupations and contexts or to evaluate occupational therapy interventions directed at individuals or populations, occupational therapy practitioners require information regarding their clients (i.e., the domains and dimensions of practice) and outcomes, as well as the type, frequency, duration, and timing of interventions. If occupational therapists routinely collect and record this information, they can use it not only to guide intervention but also to conduct research on practice. In fact, the professions that have most consistently used information gleaned in the course of providing routine care (e.g., medicine) have the largest body of evidence regarding the use, quality, and effectiveness of their services. Occupational therapy practitioners should seize every opportunity to collect information routinely during practice and use it to test hypotheses about the importance of occupation, the contribution of engagement in occupations and participation in contexts to health and wellness, and the effectiveness of occupational therapy services directed toward individuals and populations.

Because the dimensions of the occupational therapy profession's domain of practice align with the determinants of health of individuals and populations, as described in chapter 15, practitioners routinely collect information on and monitor changes in factors that contribute to health and health outcomes such as engagement in occupations that can serve as proxy measures of well-being. Therefore, client profiles should include all the data that are needed to test hypotheses regarding the factors that contribute to the health of individuals and populations and to measure the impact of occupational therapy interventions in altering health status.

Although there are many ways to collect and record data on clients and their occupations and contexts, the new terminology proposed in the *International Classification of Functioning, Disability and Health* (ICF; WHO, 2001) can be used to promote uniform documentation across practitioners, health professions, and jurisdictions. This system of classification parallels the domain and dimensions of practice defined in *Occupational Therapy Practice Framework: Domain and Process* (American Occupational Therapy Association [AOTA], 2002). Indeed, the occupational therapy leaders who conducted the conceptual work to develop this important AOTA document used WHO documents to inform their thoughts about impairments, activity limitations, and participation restrictions.

The ICF classification system can be used as a tool when collecting and recording data about persons and their occupations and contexts and can serve as a systematic coding scheme for health information systems. This information can then be used to plan and monitor intervention directed toward individuals and populations and to measure and track target outcomes. When occupational therapy practitioners document information for client profiles using either the ICF or dimensions defined in the *Occupational Therapy Practice Framework* (AOTA, 2002), these data can be used for research.

Because the ICF and the dimensions of the domain of occupational therapy practice correspond to the determinants of health defined by population health researchers, the data routinely collected by means of client profiles can be used to further test hypotheses regarding determinants of health, disability, and engagement in occupations; to understand why people with the same impairments vary in their activity limitations and partic-

CASE STUDY: CITIZEN ACTION AGAINST OBESITY

As an occupational therapy practitioner, Kim was keenly aware of her unique role within the community as a mother and as a participant in the community development process. Project partners and stakeholders who participated in the asset mapping process identified health determinants that paralleled her understanding of key contributors to the health of children and their levels of wellness as they matured.

Many of the participants had concerns about the increasing number of obese children, and they wondered about changes in nutrition and physical activity. They had heard about the impact of obesity on general health and wellness across the life span, but they could not recall the specifics of information they had received about these effects. They asked Kim to guide them through a focus group session to further explore the epidemiology of obesity and research on the impact of obesity on health across the life span. Kim suggested that once they completed their analysis of the obesity problem in their community, she could facilitate the development of a proposal to seek funds for a research initiative. The community participants were motivated to learn more and to identify opportunities to work together with children and their families to nurture and support lifestyles and environments in support of healthy body weights.

The community members learned that obesity was a more complex health condition than anticipated and epitomized the importance of considering social, behavioral, cultural, environmental, physiological, and genetic factors as determinants of health. Because overweight and obesity are major contributors to many preventable causes of poor health and death, it is among one of the 10 leading health indicators in *Healthy People 2010* (DHHS, 2000). Kim took community leaders through a process of examining the parameters of the problem as reflected in population health data. She focused on describing the characteristics of persons that predispose them to obesity, the profiles of their typical engagement in occupations and participation in contexts, and descriptions of customary environmental contexts that contribute (or not) to healthy body weights. It became apparent to the community members that prevention should target individuals who are at risk for obesity and focus on individual characteristics that are amenable to change and the environmental contexts that most influence children. One of the more immediate objectives was to conduct a survey of the physical, social, and cultural environments to learn more about how to halt the obesity epidemic in their community. Kim would coauthor the funding proposal and be the coinvestigator on the project. ■

ipation restrictions; and to determine the effectiveness of occupational therapy evaluation and intervention.

Common systems of classification lay the foundation for the establishment of a common language for describing functional states and permit aggregation and comparison of data across practitioners, health care disciplines, services, and time. Wilcock (1998) described an action research approach that can help occupational therapists make a unique contribution to population health research. This chapter provides readers the opportunity to explore the use of task analysis in a research-driven intervention to combat obesity among members of a community.

The Challenge

1. Read the case study of Citizen Action Against Obesity. Describe how task analysis was used to focus the analysis of issues facing the community, to explore research into factors that contribute to this problem, and to identify intervention options for addressing the goal of reducing the prevalence of obesity.

2. Through a library and Internet search, determine the prevalence of obesity in the United

States and identify factors that are known to influence the prevalence of obesity. Describe the characteristics of intervention approaches that appear to show results against this growing public health "epidemic."

3. Describe how you might use task analysis to enable an individual client or a group of clients who are obese to reflect on the determinants of their own health state. How might you use task analysis as a tool to guide intervention with these clients?

4. How might you use task analysis to promote the collective sharing of critical self-reflections among a group of people who are obese? Because people are often unaware of the characteristics of their customary environments that adversely influence their health, how might you use task analysis in a group context

as an educational tool? How might this participation model facilitate social action by a group or community?

5. Describe how you might use task analysis to enable a group of clients who are not obese to reflect on the determinants of obesity and opportunities they can seize to contribute to national efforts to address this public health problem. ■

Learning Resources

Centers for Disease Control and Prevention information on fetal alcohol syndrome: www.cdc.gov/ncbddd/fas

National Institute of Alcohol Abuse and Alcoholism: www.niaaa.nih.gov

National Institute of Drug Abuse: www.nida.nih.gov

Nestle, M., & Jacobson, M. F. (2000). Halting the obesity epidemic: A public health policy approach. *Public Health Reports, 115*, 12–24.

References

Abreu, B. C., & Toglia, J. P. (1987). Cognitive rehabilitation: A model of occupational therapy. *American Journal of Occupational Therapy, 41,* 439–448.

Administration on Aging. (2001). *A profile of older Americans: 2001.* Washington, DC: U.S. Department of Health and Human Services.

Aldana, S. G. (2001). Financial impact of health promotion programs: A comprehensive review of the literature. *American Journal of Health Promotion, 15,* 296–320.

American Medical Association, & U.S. Department of Health and Human Services. (2002). *A primer on population-based medicine.* Retrieved from http://www.ama-assn.org/ama/pub/category/6886.html

American Occupational Therapy Association. (1973). *The roles and functions of occupational therapy personnel.* Bethesda, MD: Author.

American Occupational Therapy Association. (1974). *A curriculum guide for occupational therapy educators.* Bethesda, MD: Author.

American Occupational Therapy Association. (1979). *Occupational therapy product output reporting system and uniform terminology for reporting occupational therapy services.* Bethesda, MD: Author.

American Occupational Therapy Association. (1991). *1990 membership data survey.* Bethesda, MD: Author.

American Occupational Therapy Association. (1993). Position paper: Purposeful activity. *American Journal of Occupational Therapy, 47,* 1081–1082.

American Occupational Therapy Association. (1994a). *Uniform terminology: Application to practice.* Bethesda, MD: Author.

American Occupational Therapy Association. (1994b). *Uniform terminology for occupational therapy* (3rd ed.). Bethesda, MD: Author.

American Occupational Therapy Association. (1995a). *Essentials and guidelines for an accredited educational program for the occupational therapist.* Bethesda, MD: Author.

American Occupational Therapy Association. (1995b). *Essentials and guidelines for an accredited educational program for the occupational therapy assistant.* Bethesda, MD: Author.

American Occupational Therapy Association. (1996). OT practitioners work more with elderly patients. *OT Practice, 1*(3), 17.

American Occupational Therapy Association. (1997). The psychosocial core of occupational therapy position paper. *American Journal of Occupational Therapy, 51,* 868–869.

American Occupational Therapy Association. (2001). Occupational therapy in the promotion of health and the prevention of disease and disability statement. *American Journal of Occupational Therapy, 55,* 656–660.

American Occupational Therapy Association. (2002). Occupational therapy practice framework: Domain and process. *American Journal of Occupational Therapy, 56,* 609–639.

Americans With Disabilities Act of 1990. Pub. L. 101–336, 42 U.S.C. § 12101.

Anderson, C., Mhurchu, C. N., Rubenach, S., Clark, M., Spencer, C., & Winsor, A. (2000). Home or hospital for stroke rehabilitation? Results of a randomized controlled trial: II. Cost minimization analysis at 6 months. *Stroke, 31,* 1032.

Assistive Technology Act of 1998. Pub. L. No. 105-394, §2, 29 Stat. 3628.

Assistive Technology Training. (2002). *Assistive technology training online project.* Retrieved from http://www.atto.buffalo.edu/printfriendly.php?filepath=/registered/ATBasics/Foundation/intro

Atwood, C. E. (1907). The favourable influence of occupation in certain nervous disorders. *New York Medical Journal, 86,* 1101–1103.

Ayres, A. J. (1979). *Sensory integration and the child.* Los Angeles: Western Psychological Service.

Bachmann, K. (2000). *More than just hard hats and safety boots: Creating healthier work environments.* Ottawa, ON: Conference Board of Canada.

Baum, C. (1998). Client-centered practice in a changing health care system. In M. Law (Ed.), *Client-centered occupational therapy* (pp. 29–46). Thorofare, NJ: Slack.

Blau, Z. (1973). *Old age in a changing society.* New York: New Viewpoints.

Bonder, B. R. (1994). The psychosocial meaning of activity. In B. R. Bonder & M. B. Wagner (Eds.), *Functional performance in older adults* (pp. 28–40). Philadelphia: F. A. Davis.

Bonder, B. R., & Goodman, G. (1995). Preventing occupational dysfunction secondary to aging. In C. A. Trombly (Ed.), *Occupational therapy for physical dysfunction* (4th ed., pp. 391–404). Baltimore: Williams & Wilkins.

Brown v. Board of Education, 347 U.S. 483 (1954).

Bundy, A. (1993). Assessment of play and leisure: Delineation of the problem. *American Journal of Occupational Therapy, 47,* 217–222.

Bureau of the Census. (1997, December). *Disabilities affect one-fifth of all Americans: Proportion will increase in coming decades* (Census Brief). Washington, DC: Author.

Bureau of the Census. (2000). *Population projections.* Washington, DC: Author.

Canadian Association of Occupational Therapists. (1991). *Canadian occupational therapy guidelines for client-centred practice.* Toronto, ON: Author.

Canadian Association of Occupational Therapists. (1993). *Occupational therapy guidelines for client-centred mental health practice.* Toronto, ON: Author.

Canadian Association of Occupational Therapists. (1997). *Enabling occupation: An occupational therapy perspective.* Ottawa, ON: Author.

Canadian Association of Occupational Therapists. (2002). Models and evidence in occupational therapy. *Canadian Journal of Occupational Therapy, 64,* 186.

Canfield, H., & Locke, B. (1996). *A book of possibilities: Activities using simple technology.* Minneapolis, MN: AbleNet.

Carnegie Council on Adolescent Development. (1995). *Great transitions: Preparing adolescents for a new century.* New York: Carnegie Corporation.

Case-Smith, J. (1991). The family perspective. In W. Dunn (Ed.), *Pediatric occupational therapy: Facilitating effective service provision* (pp. 319–332). Thorofare, NJ: Slack.

Case-Smith, J. (1996). An overview of occupational therapy for children. In J. Case-Smith, A. S. Allen, & P. N. Pratt (Eds.), *Occupational therapy for children* (3rd ed., pp. 3–17). St. Louis, MO: Mosby.

Case-Smith, J., Allen, A. S., & Pratt, P. N. (1996). *Occupational therapy for children* (3rd ed.). St. Louis, MO: Mosby.

Cavaiola, A. A. (1999). Suicidal behavior in chemically dependent adolescents. *Adolescence, 34*(136), 735–744. Abstract retrieved from http://www.findarticles.com/cf_dis/m2248/136_34/59810230/print.jhtml

Center for Applied Technology. (2002). *Universal design for living.* Retrieved from www.cast.org/udl/index.cfm?i+11

Centers for Disease Control and Prevention. (2002). *Fetal alcohol syndrome: Defining the national agendas.* Retrieved from www.cdc.gov/ncbddd/fas

Chen, J., & Millar, W. J. (2000). Are recent cohorts healthier than their predecessors? *Health Reports, 11,* 9–23.

Christiansen, C. (1999). Defining lives: Occupation as an identity—An essay on competence, coherence, and creation of meaning (1999 Eleanor Clark Slagle Lecture). *American Journal of Occupational Therapy, 53,* 547–558.

Christiansen, C., & Baum, C. (Eds.). (1991). *Occupational therapy: Overcoming human performance deficits.* Thorofare, NJ: Slack.

Christiansen, C., & Baum, C. (Eds.). (1997). *Occupational therapy: Enabling functioning and well-being* (2nd ed.). Thorofare, NJ: Slack.

Clark, F., Azen, S. P., Carlson, M., Mandel, D., LaBree, L., Hay, J., Zemke, R., Jackson, J., & Lipson, L. (2001). Embedding health-promoting changes into the daily lives of independent living older adults: Long-term follow-up of occupational therapy intervention. *Journals of Gerontology Series B: Psychological Sciences and Social Sciences, 56*(1), 60–63.

Clark, F., Azen, S. P., Zemke, R., Jackson, J., Carlson, M., Mandel, D., Hay, J., Josephson, K., Cherry, B., Hessel, C., Palmer, J., & Lipson, L. (1997). Occupational therapy for independent living older adults. *Journal of the American Medical Association, 278,* 1321–1326.

Clark, F. A., Parham, D., Carlson, M. E., Frank, G., Jackson, J., Pierce, D., Wolfe, R. J., & Zemke, R. (1991). Occupational science: Academic innovation in the science of occupational therapy's future. *American Journal of Occupational Therapy, 45,* 300–310.

Community Action Toward Children's Health. (2001). *Year 2 report: Learning to walk and talk.* Kelowna, BC: Author. (See also www.catch.silk.net)

Cook, A. M., & Hussey, S. M. (1995). *Assistive technologies: Principles and practice.* St. Louis, MO: Mosby.

Creighton, C. (1992). The origin and evolution of activity analysis. *American Journal of Occupational Therapy, 46,* 45–48.

Csikszentmihalyi, M. (1990). *Flow: The psychology of optimal experience.* New York: Harper & Row.

Cynkin, S. (1979). *Occupational therapy: Toward health through activities.* Boston: Little, Brown.

Davidson, H. (1991). Performance and the social environment. In C. Christiansen & C. Baum (Eds.), *Occupational therapy: Overcoming human performance deficits* (pp. 144–177). Thorofare, NJ: Slack.

Davis, C. M. (1989). *Patient–practitioner interaction: An experiential manual for developing the art of health care.* Thorofare, NJ: Slack.

Donohue, M. V., & Greer, E. (2000). Designing group activities to meet individual and group goals. In J. Hinojosa & M. L. Blount (Eds.), *Texture of life: Purposeful activities in occupational therapy* (pp. 159–195). Bethesda, MD: American Occupational Therapy Association.

Donovan, D. M., & McIntyre, D. (1985). *Healing the hurt child: A developmental–contextual approach.* New York: W. W. Norton.

Dow, P. W., & Rees, N. P. (1995). High technology adaptations to overcome disability. In C. A. Trombly (Ed.), *Occupational therapy for physical dysfunction* (4th ed., pp. 611–643). Baltimore: Williams & Wilkins.

Duggal, S. (2000). Assessment of life stress in adolescents: Self-report versus interview methods. *Journal of the American Academy of Child and Adolescent Psychiatry, 39,* 455–452. Abstract retrieved from www.findartcles.com/cf_dls/m2250/4_39/61909222/print.jhtml

Dunlop, W. J. (1933). A brief history of occupational therapy. *Canadian Journal of Occupational Therapy, 1,* 6–11.

Dunn, W. (1998). *Best practice occupational therapy in community service with children and families.* (2nd ed) Thorofare, NJ: Slack.

Dunn, W. (2000). *Best practice occupational therapy in community service with children and families.* (2nd ed) Thorofare, NJ: Slack.

Dunn, W., Brown, C., & McGuigan, A. (1994). The ecology of human performance: A framework for considering the effect of context. *American Journal of Occupational Therapy, 48,* 595–607.

Dunn, W., Foto, M., Hinojosa, J., Schell, B. A. B., Thomson, L. K., & Hertfelder, S. D. (1996). Occupational therapy: A profession in support of full inclusion. *American Journal of Occupational Therapy, 50,* 855.

Earls, F. (2001). Community factors supporting child mental health. *Child and Adolescent Psychiatry Clinics of North America, 10,* 693–709.

Evans, R. G., Barer, M. L., & Marmor, T. R. (Eds.). (1994). *Why are some people healthy and others not?* Hawthorne, NY: Aldine de Gruyter.

Fazio, L. S. (2001). *Developing occupation-centered programs for the community: A workbook for students and professionals.* Upper Saddle River, NJ: Prentice Hall.

Ferland, F. (1992). Le jeu en ergothé: Reflexion préable à l'élaboration d'un nouveau modèle de pratique. *Canadian Journal of Occupational Therapy, 59,* 95–101.

Fidler, G. S. (1981). From crafts to competence. *American Journal of Occupational Therapy, 35,* 567–573.

Fidler, G. S., & Fidler, J. (1978). Doing and becoming: Purposeful action and self-actualization. *American*

Journal of Occupational Therapy, 32, 305–310.

Fisher, A. (1995). Successful aging, life satisfaction, and generativity in later life. *International Journal of Aging and Human Development, 41,* 239–250.

Fisher, A., & Kielhofner, G. (1995). Skill in occupational performance. In G. Kielhofner (Ed.), *A model of human occupation: Theory and application* (2nd ed., pp. 113–128). Philadelphia: Lippincott, Williams & Wilkins.

Flemming, M. (1994). A common sense practice in an uncommon world. In C. Mattingly & M. H. Flemming (Eds.), *Clinical reasoning: Forms of inquiry in a therapeutic practice* (pp. 94–116). Philadelphia: F. A. Davis.

Florey, L. (1998). Psychosocial dysfunction in childhood and adolescence. In M. E. Neistadt & E. B. Crepeau (Eds.), *Willard & Spackman's occupational therapy* (9th ed., pp. 622–635). Philadelphia: Lippincott.

Floyd, R. I., Decoufle, P., & Hungerford, D. W. (1999). Alcohol use prior to pregnancy recognition. *American Journal of Preventive Medicine, 17,* 101–107.

Forer, S. (1996). *Outcome management and program evaluation made easy: A toolkit for occupational therapy practitioners.* Bethesda, MD: American Occupational Therapy Association.

Forsyth, K., & Kielhofner, G. (1999). Validity of the assessment of communication of interaction skills. *British Journal of Occupational Therapy, 62,* 69–74.

Forsyth, K., Salamy, M., Simon, S., & Kielhofner, G. (1997). *Assessment of communication and interaction skills.* Chicago: University of Illinois, Model of Human Occupation Clearinghouse.

Frank, G. (1996a). Life histories in occupational therapy practice. *American Journal of Occupational Therapy, 50,* 251–264.

Frank, G. (1996b). The concept of adaptation as a foundation for occupational science research. In R. Zemke & F. Clark (Eds.), *Occupational science: The evolving discipline* (pp. 47–55). Philadelphia: F. A. Davis.

Friedland, J. (2001). Knowing from where we came: Reflecting on return-to-work and interpersonal relationships. *Canadian Journal of Occupational Therapy, 68,* 266–271.

Friedman, H. M. (1916, September 23). Occupational specialization in the defective. *New York Medical Journal,* pp. 587–592.

Fries, J. F. (1983). The compression of morbidity. *Milbank Quarterly, 61,* 397–419.

Gage, M. (1992). The appraisal model of coping: An

assessment and intervention model for occupational therapy. *American Journal of Occupational Therapy, 46,* 353–362.

Gage, M., & Polatajko, H. (1994). Enhancing occupational performance through an understanding of perceived self-efficacy. *American Journal of Occupational Therapy, 48,* 452–461.

Gilbreth, F. B. (1911). *Motion study.* New York: Nostrand.

Glanz, K., Lewis, F. M., & Rimer, B. K. (Eds.). (1997). *Health behavior and health education: Theory, research, and practice.* San Francisco: Jossey-Bass.

Glickman, L., Deitz, J., Anson, D., & Stewart, K. (1996). The effect of switch control site on computer skills of infants and toddlers. *American Journal of Occupational Therapy, 50,* 545–553.

Gorski, G., & Miyake, S. (1985). The adolescent life/work planning group: A prevention model. *Occupational Therapy in Health Care, 2*(3), 139–150.

Graham-Berman, S. A., Coupet, S., Egler, L., Mattis, J., & Banyard, V. (1996). Interpersonal relationships and adjustment of children in homeless and economically stressed families. *Journal of Clinical Child Psychology, 25,* 250–261.

Gray, D. B., & Hahn, H. (1997). Achieving occupational goals. In C. H. Christiansen & C. M. Baum (Eds.), *Occupational therapy: Enabling function and well-being* (2nd ed., pp. 392–409). Thorofare, NJ: Slack.

Green, L. W., & Kreuter, M. W. (1999). *Health promotion planning: An educational and ecological approach* (3rd ed.). Mountain View, CA: Mayfield.

Haas, L. J. (1922). Crafts adaptable to occupational need: Their relative importance. *Archives of Occupational Therapy, 1,* 443–445.

Hagedorn, R. (1997). *Foundations for practice in occupational therapy.* New York: Churchill Livingstone.

Hall, H. J. (1910). The work cure. *Journal of the American Medical Association, 54,* 12.

Hall, H. J. (1922). Occupational therapy in 1921. *Modern Hospital, 18,* 61–63.

Hamilton, B. B., Granger, C. V., Sherwin, F. S., Zielezny, M., & Tashman, J. S. (1987). A uniform national data system for medical rehabilitation. In M. J. Fuhrer (Ed.), *Rehabilitation outcomes: Analysis and measurement* (pp. 125–147). Baltimore: Paul H. Brookes.

Hansen, C. (1999). ADHD boys in young adulthood: Psychosocial adjustment. *Journal of the American Academy of Child and Adolescent Psychiatry.* Retrieved from http://www.findarticles.com/cf_dis/m2250/2_38/54035849/print.jhtml

Hasselkus, B. R. (1998). Introduction to adult and older populations. In M. E. Neistadt & E. B. Crepeau (Eds.), *Willard & Spackman's occupational therapy* (9th ed., pp. 651–659). Philadelphia: Lippincott.

Hauser, S. T., Borman, E. H., Powers, S. I., Jacobson, A. M., & Noam, G. G. (1990). Paths of adolescent ego development: Links with family life and individual adjustment. *Psychiatric Clinics of North America, 13,* 489–510.

Hawking, S. W. (1996). Striving for excellence in the presence of disabilities. In R. Zemke & F. Clark (Eds.), *Occupational science: The evolving discipline* (pp. 27–30). Philadelphia: F. A. Davis.

Hay, J., Labree, L., Luo, R., Clark, F., Carlson, M., Mandel, D., Zemke, R., Jackson, J., & Azen, S. P. (2002). Cost-effectiveness of preventive occupational therapy for independent living older adults. *Journal of the American Geriatrics Society, 50,* 1381–1387.

Heaney, C. A., & Goetzel, R. Z. (1997). A review of health-related outcomes of multi-component worksite health promotion programs. *American Journal of Health Promotion, 11,* 290–307.

Heckman, J. (2000). *Policies to foster human capital.* Chicago: University of Chicago Press.

Helfrich, C., & Kielhofner, G. (1994). Volitional narratives and the meaning of therapy. *American Journal of Occupational Therapy, 48,* 326.

Helfrich, C., Kielhofner, G., & Mattingly, C. (1994). Volition as narrative: Understanding motivation in chronic illness. *American Journal of Occupational Therapy, 48,* 311–317.

Henry, A. D. (1998). The interview process in occupational therapy. In M. E. Neistadt & E. B. Crepeau (Eds.), *Willard & Spackman's occupational therapy* (9th ed., pp. 155–167). Philadelphia: Lippincott.

Hess, K. A., & Campion, E. W. (1983). Motivating the geriatric patient for rehabilitation. *Journal of the American Geriatric Society, 31,* 586–589.

Hinojosa, J., Sabari, J., & Rosenfeld, M. S. (1983). Purposeful activities. *American Journal of Occupational Therapy, 37,* 805–806.

Hislop, H. J., & Montgomery, J. (1995). *Daniels and Worthingham's muscle testing: Techniques of manual examination* (6th ed.). Philadelphia: Saunders.

Hopkins, H. L. (1988). *An historical perspective on*

occupational therapy. In H. L. Hopkins & H. D. Smith (Eds.), *Willard & Spackman's occupational therapy.* Philadelphia: Lippincott.

Hsieh, C., Nelson, D. L., Smith, D. A., & Peterson, C. Q. (1996). A comparison of performance in added-purpose occupations and rote exercise for dynamic standing balance in persons with hemiplegia. *American Journal of Occupational Therapy, 50,* 10–16.

Individuals With Disabilities Education Act of 1990. Pub. L. 101–476, 20 U.S.C., Ch. 33.

Jackson, J., Carlson, M., Mandel, D., Zemke, R., & Clark, F. (1998). Occupation in lifestyle redesign: The well elderly study occupational therapy program. *American Journal of Occupational Therapy, 52,* 326–336.

Jackson, J., Mandel, D. R., Zemke, R., & Clark, F. A. (2001). Promoting quality of life in elders: An occupation-based occupational therapy program. *World Federation of Occupational Therapists Bulletin, 43,* 5–12.

Kaufman, M. (1990). *Nutrition in public health: A handbook for developing programs and services.* Gaithersburg, MD: Aspen.

Kaye, H. S. (1997). *Education of children with disabilities* (Disability Statistics Abstract 19). Washington, DC: U.S. Department of Education, National Institute on Disability and Rehabilitation Research.

Kaye, H. S. (1998). *Is the status of people with disabilities improving?* (Disability Statistics Abstract Report 21). Washington, DC: U.S. Department of Education, National Institute on Disability and Rehabilitation Research.

Kaye, H. S. (2000). *Computer and Internet use among people with disabilities* (Disability Statistics Report 13). Washington, DC: U.S. Department of Education, National Institute on Disability and Rehabilitation Research.

Kenny, M. E. (1996). Promoting optimal adolescent development from a developmental and contextual framework. *Counseling Psychologist, 24,* 475–481.

Kidner, T. B. (1923). President's address. *Archives of Occupational Therapy, 2,* 415–424.

Kidner, T. B. (1930). *Occupational therapy: The science of prescribed work for invalids.* Stuttgart, Germany: W. Kohlhammer.

Kielhofner, G. (1985). *A model of human occupation: Theory and application.* Baltimore: Williams & Wilkins.

Kielhofner, G. (1995). *A model of human occupation: Theory and application* (2nd ed.). Baltimore:

Williams & Wilkins.

Kielhofner, G. (1997). *Conceptual foundations of occupational therapy* (2nd ed.). Philadelphia: F. A. Davis.

King, L. J. (1978). Toward a science of adaptive responses (1978 Eleanor Clarke Slagle Lecture). *American Journal of Occupational Therapy, 32,* 429–437.

Kirscher, M. A. (1984). Motivation as a factor of perceived exertion in purposeful versus nonpurposeful activity. *American Journal of Occupational Therapy, 38,* 165–170.

Labonte, R. (1993). *Health promotion and empowerment: Practice frameworks.* Toronto, ON: University of Toronto.

LaPlante, M. P., Carlson, D., Kaye, H. S., & Bradsher, J. E. (1996). *Families with disabilities in the United States* (Disability Statistics Reports 8). Washington, DC: U.S. Department of Education, National Institute on Disability and Rehabilitation Research.

Larson, K. O., Stevens-Ratchford, R. G., Pedretti, L., & Crabtree, J. L. (1996). *The role of occupational therapy with the elderly,* (2nd ed.). Bethesda, MD: American Occupational Therapy Association.

Law, M. (2002a). Participation in the occupations of everyday life. *American Journal of Occupational Therapy, 56,* 640–649.

Law, M. (Ed.). (2002b). *Evidence-based rehabilitation: A guide to practice.* Thorofare, NJ: Slack.

Law, M., Cooper, B., Strong, S., Stewart, D., Rigby, P., & Letts, L. (1996). The person–environment–occupation model: A transactive approach to occupational performance. *Canadian Journal of Occupational Therapy, 63,* 9–23.

Law, M., Polatajko, H., Baptiste, W., & Townsend, E. (1997). Core concepts of occupational therapy. In Canadian Association of Occupational Therapists (Ed.), *Enabling occupation: An occupational therapy perspective* (pp. 29–56). Ottawa, ON: Canadian Association of Occupational Therapists.

Letts, L., Law, M., Rigby, P., Cooper, B., Stewart, D., & Strong, S. (1994). Person–environment assessments in occupational therapy. *American Journal of Occupational Therapy, 48,* 608–618.

Lewin, J. E., & Reed, C. A. (1998). *Creative problem solving in occupational therapy: With stories about children.* Philadelphia: Lippincott.

Licht, B. C., & Nelson, D. L. (1990). Adding meaning to a design copy task through representational stimuli. *American Journal of Occupational Therapy,*

44, 408–413.

Mandel, D. R., Jackson, J., Zemke, R., Nelson, L., & Clark, F. (1999). *Lifestyle redesign: Implementing the well-elderly program.* Bethesda, MD: American Occupational Therapy Association.

Mattingly, C., & Flemming, M. H. (1994). *Clinical reasoning: Forms of inquiry in therapeutic practice.* Philadelphia: F. A. Davis.

May, P. A., & Gossage, J. P. (2001). Estimating the prevalence of fetal alcohol syndrome: A summary. *Alcohol Research & Health, 25,* 159–167.

Mayberry, W. (1990). Self-esteem in children: Considerations for measurement and intervention. *American Journal of Occupational Therapy, 44,* 729–734.

McBeth, A. J., & Schweer, K. D. (Eds.). (2000). *Building healthy communities.* Boston: Allyn & Bacon.

McHale, K., & Cermak, S. A. (1992). Fine motor activities in elementary school: Preliminary findings and provisional implications for children with fine motor problems. *American Journal of Occupational Therapy, 46,* 898–903.

McKenzie, J. F., & Smeltzer, J. L. (2001). *Planning, implementing, and evaluating health promotion programs: A primer* (3rd ed.). Boston: Allyn & Bacon.

McNeil, J. M. (1993). *Americans with disabilities: 1991–1992* (Current Population Reports P70-33). Washington, DC: U.S. Government Printing Office.

McNeil, J. M. (1997). Americans with disabilities: 1994–95. U.S. Bureau of the Census, Current Population Reports, P70-61. Washington, DC: U.S. Department of Commerce.

McNeil, J. (2001). *Americans with disabilities: Household economic studies.* Washington, DC: Bureau of the Census.

McNeil, J. M., Lamas, E. J., & Harpine, C. J. (1986). *Disability, functional limitation, and health insurance coverage.* Washington, DC: U.S. Government Printing Office.

Menec, V., MacWilliam, L., Soodeen, R., & Mitchell, L. (2002). *The health and health care use of Manitoba's seniors: Have they changed over time?* Winnipeg, MB: Manitoba Centre for Health Policy.

Meyer, A. (1922). The philosophy of occupational therapy. *Archives of Occupational Therapy, 1,* 1–10.

Mistrett, S. G., & Lane, S. J. (1995). Using assistive technology for play and learning: Children, from birth to 10 years of age. In W. Mann & J. Lane (Eds.), *Assistive technology for persons with dis-*

ability (4th ed.) (pp. 131–163). Bethesda, MD: American Occupational Therapy Association.

Moher, T. J. (1907). Occupation in the treatment of the insane. *Journal of the American Medical Association, 158,* 1664–1666.

Mosey, A. C. (1981). *Occupational therapy: Configuration of a profession.* New York: Raven Press.

Mosey, A. C. (1986). *Psychosocial components of occupational therapy.* New York: Raven Press.

Mosey, A. C. (1996). *Applied scientific inquiry in health professions: An epidemiological orientation* (2nd ed.). Bethesda, MD: American Occupational Therapy Association.

Moyers, P. A. (1999). Guide to occupational therapy practice. *American Journal of Occupational Therapy, 53,* 248–322.

National Institute for Occupational Safety and Health. (2002). *Traumatic occupational injuries.* Retrieved from http://www.cdc.gov/niosh/injury/trauma.html

National Institute of Mental Health. (2001). *Older adults: Depression and suicide facts.* Bethesda, MD: Author. (See also www.nimh.nih.gov/publicat/elderlydepsuicide.pdf)

National Mental Health Association. (2002). *Depression and older Americans.* Retrieved from http://www.hmha.org/ccd/support/factsheet.older.cfm

Neistadt, M. E. (1998). Introduction to evaluation and interviewing. In M. E. Neistadt & E. B. Crepeau (Eds.), *Willard & Spackman's occupational therapy* (9th ed., pp. 151–155). Philadelphia: Lippincott.

Neistadt, M. E., & Crepeau, E. B. (Eds.). (1998). *Willard & Spackman's occupational therapy* (9th ed.). Philadelphia: Lippincott.

Nestle, M., & Jacobson, M. F. (2000). Halting the obesity epidemic: A public health policy approach. *Public Health Reports, 115,* 12–24.

O'Donnell, M. P. (1989). Definition of health promotion: Part III. Expanding the definition. *American Journal of Health Promotion, 3,* 5.

O'Donnell, M. P. (2000). *How to design workplace health promotion programs.* Keego, MI: American Journal of Health Promotion.

Organisation for Economic Co-operation and Development. (2001). *Starting strong: Early childhood education and care.* Paris: Author. (See also www.childcarecanada.org/policy/polstudies/int/OECDstrong.html)

Pan American Health Organization. (2002). *Healthy municipalities and communities.* Retrieved from www.paho.org/English/HPP/HPF/HMC/hmc_about.htm

Parham, L. D., & Fazio, L. S. (1997). *Play in occupational therapy for children.* St. Louis, MO: Mosby.

Pasek, P. B., & Schkade, J. K. (1996). Effects of skiing experiences on adolescents with limb deficiencies: An occupational adaptation perspective. *American Journal of Occupational Therapy, 50,* 24–31.

Pelletier, K. R. (2001). A review and analysis of the clinical- and cost-effectiveness studies of comprehensive health promotion and disease management programs at the worksite: 1998–2000 update. *American Journal of Health Promotion, 16,* 107–116.

Peterson, A. C. (1993). Creating adolescents: The role of context and process in developmental trajectories (Presidential Address). *Journal of Research on Adolescence, 3*(1), 1–18.

Pierce, D. (2001). Untangling occupation and activity. *American Journal of Occupational Therapy, 55,* 138–146.

Polatajko, H. J. (1992). Naming and framing occupational therapy: A lecture dedicated to the life of Nancy B. *Canadian Journal of Occupational Therapy, 59,* 184–200.

Polatajko, H. J. (1994). Dreams, dilemmas, and decisions for occupational therapy practice in the new millennium: A Canadian perspective. *American Journal of Occupational Therapy, 48,* 590–594.

Polatajko, H. J. (2001). The evolution of our occupational perspective: The journey from diversion through therapeutic use to enablement. *Canadian Journal of Occupational Therapy, 68,* 203–207.

Polkinghorne, D. E. (1996). Transformative narratives: From victim to agentic life plots. *American Journal of Occupational Therapy, 50,* 299–305.

Price-Lankey, P., & Cashman, J. (1996). Jenny's story: Reinventing oneself through occupation and narrative configuration. *American Journal of Occupational Therapy, 50,* 306–314.

Public Health Foundation. (2002). *Healthy people 2010 toolkit.* Washington, DC: Author. (See also www.health. gov/healthypeople/state/toolkit)

Puska, P., Tuomilehto, J., Nissinen, A., & Vartiainen, E. (1995). *The North Karelia Project: 20-year results and experiences.* Finland: National Public Health Institute, KTL.

Quintana, L. (1995). Evaluation of perception and cognition. In C. A. Trombly (Ed.), *Occupational therapy for physical dysfunction* (pp. 201–224). Baltimore: Williams & Wilkins.

Raeburn, J., & Rootman, I. (1998). *People-centered health promotion.* Toronto, ON: Wiley.

Reed, K. L. (1998). Theory and frame of reference. In M. E. Neistadt & E. B. Crepeau (Eds.), *Willard & Spackman's occupational therapy* (9th ed., pp. 521–524). Philadelphia: Lippincott.

Reilly, M. (1974). *Play as exploratory learning: Studies in curiosity behavior.* Beverly Hills, CA: Sage.

Remen, R. N. (1996). *Kitchen table wisdom.* New York: Riverhead Books.

Rogers, J., & Holm, M. (1994). Assessment of self care. In B. R. Bonder & M. B. Wagner (Eds.), *Functional performance in older adults* (pp. 181–202). Philadelphia: F. A. Davis.

Ross, N. A., Wolfson, M. C., Dunn, J. R., Bethelot, J. M., Kaplan, G. A., & Lynch, J. W. (2000). Relation between income inequality and mortality in Canada and in the United States: Cross-sectional assessment using census data and vital statistics. *British Medical Journal, 320,* 898–902.

Rowe, J. W., & Kahn, R. L. (1998). *Successful aging.* New York: Pantheon Books.

Rutters, M. (1995). *Psychosocial disturbances in young people: Challenges for prevention.* Cambridge, MA: Cambridge University Press.

Sabonis-Chafee, B., & Hussey, S. M. (1998). *Introduction to occupational therapy* (2nd ed.). St. Louis, MO: Mosby.

Schwartzberg, S. L. (1998). Group process. In M. E. Neistadt & E. B. Crepeau (Eds.), *Willard & Spackman's occupational therapy* (9th ed., pp. 120–132). Philadelphia: Lippincott.

Shalala, D. (2000). In U.S. Department of Health and Human Services, *Healthy people 2010: Understanding and improving health.* Washington, DC: Department of Health and Human Services.

Shortridge, S. D. (1989). The developmental process: Prenatal to adolescence. In P. N. Pratt & A. S. Allen (Eds.), *Occupational therapy for children* (pp. 48–64). St. Louis, MO: Mosby.

Shuster, N. (1993). Addressing assistive technology needs in special education. *American Journal of Occupational Therapy, 47,* 993–997.

Smith, R. O. (1991). Technological approaches to performance enhancement. In C. Christiansen & C. Baum (Eds.), *Occupational therapy: Overcoming human performance deficits* (pp. 747–788). Thorofare, NJ: Slack.

Spencer, J. C. (1998). Evaluation of performance contexts. In M. E. Neistadt & E. B. Crepeau (Eds.),

Willard & Spackman's occupational therapy (9th ed., pp. 291–310). Philadelphia: Lippincott.

Steinberg, L. (1998). Adolescence. In *Gale Encyclopedia of Childhood and Adolescence*. Abstract retrieved from www.findarticles.com/cf_dls/g2602/0000/2602000013/print.jhtml

Stepanek, K. M. J. T. (2000). *Journey through heartsongs*. Alexandria, VA: VSP Books.

Stotts, K. M. (1986). Health maintenance: Paraplegic athletes and non-athletes. *Archives of Physical Medicine and Rehabilitation, 67,* 109–114.

Swinth, Y. (1996). Evaluating toddlers for assistive technology. *OT Practice, 1*(3), 32–41.

Swinth, Y., Anson, D., & Deitz, J. (1993). Single-switch computer access for infants and toddlers. *American Journal for Occupational Therapy, 47,* 1031–1038.

Taylor, L. P. S., & McGruder, J. E. (1996). The meaning of sea kayaking for persons with spinal cord injuries. *American Journal of Occupational Therapy, 50,* 39–46.

Thibodeaux, C. S., & Ludwig, R. F. (1988). Intrinsic motivation in product-oriented and non-product-oriented activities. *American Journal of Occupational Therapy, 42,* 169–175.

Trombly, C. A. (1995a). Occupation: Purposefulness and meaningfulness as therapeutic mechanisms. *American Journal of Occupational Therapy, 49,* 960–972.

Trombly, C. A. (1995b). Purposeful activity. In C. A. Trombly (Ed.), *Occupational therapy for physical dysfunction* (pp. 237–253). Baltimore: Williams & Wilkins.

UNICEF. (2001). *The state of the world's children.* New York: Author. (See also www.unicef.org/sowc01/index.html)

U.S. Department of Health and Human Services. (1979). *Healthy people: The Surgeon General's report on health promotion and disease prevention.* Washington, DC: U.S. Government Printing Office.

U.S. Department of Health and Human Services. (1998). *Healthy people 2010 objectives: Draft for public comment.* Washington, DC: Author.

U.S. Department of Health and Human Services. (2000). *Healthy people 2010: Understanding and improving health.* Washington, DC: Author. (See also www.health.gov/healthypeople)

U.S. Department of Health and Human Services. (2001). *Healthy people in healthy communities: A community planning guide using Healthy People 2010.* Rockville, MD: Author. (See also www.health.gov/healthypeople/Publications/HealthyCommunities2001/default.htm)

U.S. Department of Labor. (2002). *Workplace injuries and illnesses in 2001* (News: Bureau of Labor Statistics). Washington DC: Author.

Valliant, P. M., Bezzubyk, I., Daley, L., & Asu, M. E. (1985). Psychological impact of sport on disabled athletes. *Psychological Reports, 56,* 923–929.

Van Leit, B. (1995). Using the case method to develop clinical reasoning skills in problem-based learning. *American Journal of Occupational Therapy, 49,* 349–353.

Versluys, H. P. (1995). Facilitating psychosocial adjustment to disability. In C. A. Trombly (Ed.), *Occupational therapy for physical dysfunction* (4th ed., pp. 377–389). Baltimore: Williams & Wilkins.

Wallerstein, N. (1992). Powerlessness, empowerment, and health: Implications for health promotion programs. *American Journal of Health Promotion, 6,* 197–205.

Watson, D. E. (1997). *Task analysis: An occupational performance approach.* Bethesda, MD: American Occupational Therapy Association.

Watson, D. E. (2000). *Evaluating costs and outcomes: Demonstrating the value of rehabilitation services.* Bethesda, MD: American Occupational Therapy Association.

Wheatley, C. (1996). Evaluation and treatment of cognitive dysfunction. In L. W. Pedretti (Ed.), *Occupational therapy: Practice skills for physical dysfunction* (pp. 241–252). St. Louis, MO: Mosby.

Wilcock, A. A. (1998). *An occupational perspective of health.* Thorofare, NJ: Slack.

Willoughby, C., King, G., & Polatajko, H. J. (1996). A therapist's guide to children's self-esteem. *American Journal of Occupational Therapy, 50,* 124–132.

Wilson, M. G., DeJoy, D. M., Jorgensen, C. M., & Crump, C. J. (1999). Health promotion programs in small worksites: Results of a national survey. *American Journal of Health Promotion, 13,* 358–365.

World Health Organization. (1948). Preamble to the *Constitution of the World Health Organization* as adopted by the International Health Conference, New York, 19–22 June, 1946; signed on 22 July 1946 by the representatives of 61 states (Official Records of the World Health Organization, no. 2, p. 100) and entered into force on 7 April 1948.

World Health Organization. (1980). *International classification of impairments, disabilities, and handicaps: A manual of classification relating to the consequences of disease.* Geneva, Switzerland: Author.

World Health Organization. (1984). *The health burden of social inequities.* Copenhagen, Denmark: WHO Regional Office for Europe.

World Health Organization. (1986). *The Ottawa charter for health promotion.* Ottawa, ON: Health and Welfare Canada and Author. (See also www.who.int/hpr/archive/ docs/Ottawa.html)

World Health Organization. (1998). *New players for a new era: Leading health promotion into the 21st century* (Fourth International Conference on Health Promotion, Conference Report). Geneva: Author.

World Health Organization. (2000). *Obesity: Preventing and managing the global epidemic* (Report of a WHO Consultation, WHO Tech. Rep. Series 894). Geneva, Switzerland: Author.

World Health Organization. (2001). *International classification of functioning, disability and health (ICF).* Geneva, Switzerland: Author.

Yerxa, E. J., & Baum, S. (1986). Engagement in daily occupations and life satisfaction among people with spinal cord injuries. *Occupational Therapy Journal of Research, 6,* 271–283.

Young, M. E. (2002). *From early child development to human development.* Washington, DC: World Bank. (See also www.worldbank.org/children/ECDtoHumanDevelopment.pdf)

Youngstrom, M. J. (2002). The occupational therapy practice framework: The evolution of our professional language. *American Journal of Occupational Therapy, 56,* 607–608.

Yuen, H. K. (1988). *The purposeful use of an object in the development of skill with a prosthesis.* Unpublished master's thesis, Western Michigan University, Kalamazoo.

Zahn-Waxler, C. (1996). Environment, biology, and culture: Implications for adolescent development. *Developmental Psychology, 32,* 571–573.

Zemke, R., & Clark, F. (Eds.). (1996). *Occupational science: The evolving discipline.* Philadelphia: F. A. Davis.

Appendixes

Appendix A. Areas of Occupation

Various kinds of life activities in which people engage, including ADL, IADL, education, work, play, leisure, and social participation.

■ ACTIVITIES OF DAILY LIVING (ADL)

Activities that are oriented toward taking care of one's own body (adapted from Rogers & Holm, 1994, pp. 181–202)—also called basic activities of daily living (BADL) or personal activities of daily living (PADL).

- **Bathing, showering**—Obtaining and using supplies; soaping, rinsing, and drying body parts; maintaining bathing position; and transferring to and from bathing positions.

- **Bowel and bladder management**— Includes complete intentional control of bowel movements and urinary bladder and, if necessary, use of equipment or agents for bladder control (Uniform Data System for Medical Rehabilitation [UDSMR], 1996, pp. III–20, III–24).

- **Dressing**—Selecting clothing and accessories appropriate to time of day, weather, and occasion; obtaining clothing from storage area; dressing and undressing in a sequential fashion; fastening and adjusting clothing and shoes; and applying and removing personal devices, prostheses, or orthoses.

- **Eating**—"The ability to keep and manipulate food/fluid in the mouth and swallow it" (O'Sullivan, 1995, p. 191) (AOTA, 2000, p. 629).

- **Feeding**—"The process of [setting up, arranging, and] bringing food [fluids] from the plate or cup to the mouth" (O'Sullivan, 1995, p. 191) (AOTA, 2000, p. 629).

- **Functional mobility**—Moving from one position or place to another (during performance of everyday activities), such as in-bed mobility, wheelchair mobility, transfers (wheelchair, bed, car, tub, toilet, tub/shower, chair, floor). Performing functional ambulation and transporting objects.

- **Personal device care**—Using, cleaning, and maintaining personal care items, such as hearing aids, contact lenses, glasses, orthotics, prosthetics, adaptive equipment, and contraceptive and sexual devices.

- **Personal hygiene and grooming**—Obtaining and using supplies; removing body hair (use of razors, tweezers, lotions, etc.); applying and removing cosmetics; washing, drying, combing, styling, brushing, and trimming hair; caring for nails (hands and feet); caring for skin, ears, eyes, and nose; applying deodorant; cleaning mouth; brushing and flossing teeth; or removing, cleaning, and reinserting dental orthotics and prosthetics.

- **Sexual activity**—Engagement in activities that result in sexual satisfaction.

- **Sleep/rest**—A period of inactivity in which one may or may not suspend consciousness.

- **Toilet hygiene**—Obtaining and using supplies; clothing management; maintaining toileting position; transferring to and from toileting position; cleaning body; and caring for menstrual and continence needs (including catheters, colostomies, and suppository management).

■ INSTRUMENTAL ACTIVITIES OF DAILY LIVING (IADL)

Activities that are oriented toward interacting with the environment and that are often complex—generally optional in nature (i.e., may be delegated to another) (adapted from Rogers & Holm, 1994, pp. 181–202).

- **Care of others (including selecting and supervising caregivers)**—Arranging, supervising, or providing the care for others.

- **Care of pets**—Arranging, supervising, or providing the care for pets and service animals.

- **Child rearing**—Providing the care and supervision to support the developmental needs of a child.

- **Communication device use**—Using equipment or systems such as writing equipment, telephones, typewriters, computers, communication boards, call lights, emergency systems, braille writers, telecommunication devices for the deaf, and augmentative communication systems to send and receive information.

- **Community mobility**—Moving self in the community and using public or private transportation, such as driving, or accessing buses, taxi cabs, or other public transportation systems.

- **Financial management**—Using fiscal resources, including alternate methods of financial transaction and planning and using finances with long-term and short-term goals.

- **Health management and maintenance**—Developing, managing, and maintaining routines for health and wellness promotion, such as physical fitness, nutrition, decreasing health risk behaviors, and medication routines.

- **Home establishment and management**—Obtaining and maintaining personal and household possessions and environment (e.g., home, yard, garden, appliances, vehicles), including maintaining and repairing personal possessions (clothing and household items) and knowing how to seek help or whom to contact.

- **Meal preparation and cleanup**—Planning, preparing, serving well-balanced, nutritional meals and cleaning up food and utensils after meals.

- **Safety procedures and emergency responses**—Knowing and performing preventive procedures to maintain a safe environment as well as recognizing sudden, unexpected hazardous situations and initiating emergency action to reduce the threat to health and safety.

- **Shopping**—Preparing shopping lists (grocery and other); selecting and purchasing items; selecting method of payment; and completing money transactions.

■ EDUCATION

Includes activities needed for being a student and participating in a learning environment.

- **Exploration of informal personal educational needs or interests (beyond formal education)**—Identifying topics and methods for obtaining topic-related information or skills.

- **Formal educational participation**—Including the categories of academic (e.g., math, reading, working on a degree), nonacademic (e.g., recess, lunchroom, hallway), extracurricular (e.g., sports, band, cheerleading, dances), and vocational (prevocational and vocational) participation.

- **Informal personal education participation**—Participating in classes, programs, and activities that provide instruction/training in identified areas of interest.

■ WORK

Includes activities needed for engaging in remunerative employment or volunteer activities (Mosey, 1996, p. 341).

- **Employment interests and pursuits**—Identifying and selecting work opportunities based on personal assets, limitations, likes, and dislikes relative to work (adapted from Mosey, 1996, p. 342).

- **Employment seeking and acquisition**—Identifying job opportunities, completing and submitting appropriate application materials, preparing for interviews, participating in interviews and following up afterward, discussing job benefits, and finalizing negotiations.

- **Job performance**—Including work habits, for example, attendance, punctuality, appropriate relationships with coworkers and supervisors, completion of assigned work, and compliance with the norms of the work setting (adapted from Mosey, 1996, p. 342).

- **Retirement preparation and adjustment**—Determining aptitudes, developing interests and skills, and selecting appropriate avocational pursuits.

(Continued)

Appendix A. Areas of Occupation
(Continued)

- **Volunteer exploration**—Determining community causes, organizations, or opportunities for unpaid "work" in relationship to personal skills, interests, location, and time available.

- **Volunteer participation**—Performing unpaid "work" activities for the benefit of identified selected causes, organizations, or facilities.

▨ PLAY

"Any spontaneous or organized activity that provides enjoyment, entertainment, amusement, or diversion" (Parham & Fazio, 1997, p. 252).

- **Play exploration**—Identifying appropriate play activities, which can include exploration play, practice play, pretend play, games with rules, constructive play, and symbolic play (adapted from Bergen, 1988, pp. 64–65).

- **Play participation**—Participating in play; maintaining a balance of play with other areas of occupation; and obtaining, using, and maintaining, toys, equipment, and supplies appropriately.

▨ LEISURE

"A nonobligatory activity that is intrinsically motivated and engaged in during discretionary time, that is, time not committed to obligatory occupations such as work, self-care, or sleep" (Parham & Fazio, 1997, p. 250).

- **Leisure exploration**—Identifying interests, skills, opportunities, and appropriate leisure activities.

- **Leisure participation**—Planning and participating in appropriate leisure activities; maintaining a balance of leisure activities with other areas of occupation; and obtaining, using, and maintaining equipment and supplies as appropriate.

▨ SOCIAL PARTICIPATION

Activities associated with organized patterns of behavior that are characteristic and expected of an individual or an individual interacting with others within a given social system (adapted from Mosey, 1996, p. 340).

- **Community**—Activities that result in successful interaction at the community level (i.e., neighborhood, organizations, work, school).

- **Family**—"[Activities that result in] successful interaction in specific required and/or desired familial roles" (Mosey, 1996, p. 340).

- **Peer, friend**—Activities at different levels of intimacy, including engaging in desired sexual activity.

Note. Some of the terms used in this table are from, or adapted from, the rescinded *Uniform Terminology for Occupational Therapy—Third Edition* (AOTA, 1994b, pp. 1047–1054). From *Occupational therapy practice framework: Domain and process*, by AOTA, 2002, in *American Journal of Occupational Therapy, 56*, 620–621. Reprinted with permission.

Appendix B. Performance Skills

Features of what one does, not what one has, related to observable elements of action that have implicit functional purposes (adapted from Fisher & Kielhofner, 1995, p. 113).

▨ MOTOR SKILLS
—Skills in moving and interacting with task, objects, and environment (A. Fisher, personal communication, July 9, 2001).

- **Posture**—Relates to the stabilizing and aligning of one's body while moving in relation to task objects with which one must deal.

    Stabilizes—Maintains trunk control and balance while interacting with task objects such that there is no evidence of transient (i.e., quickly passing) propping or loss of balance that affects task performance.

    Aligns—Maintains an upright sitting or standing position, without evidence of a need to persistently prop during the task performance.

    Positions—Positions body, arms, or wheelchair in relation to task objects and in a manner that promotes the use of efficient arm movements during task performance.

- **Mobility**—Relates to moving the entire body or a body part in space as necessary when interacting with task objects.

    Walks—Ambulates on level surfaces and changes direction while walking without shuffling the feet, lurching, instability, or using external supports or assistive devices (e.g., cane, walker, wheelchair) during the task performance.

    Reaches—Extends, moves the arm (and when appropriate, the trunk) to effectively grasp or place task objects that are out of reach, including skillfully using a reacher to obtain task objects.

    Bends—Actively flexes, rotates, or twists the trunk in a manner and direction appropriate to the task.

- **Coordination**—Relates to using more than one body part to interact with task objects in a manner that supports task performance.

    Coordinates—Uses two or more body parts together to stabilize and manipulate task objects during bilateral motor tasks.

    Manipulates—Uses dexterous grasp-and-release patterns, isolated finger movements, and coordinated in-hand manipulation patterns when interacting with task objects.

    Flows—Uses smooth and fluid arm and hand movements when interacting with task objects.

- **Strength and effort**—Pertains to skills that require generation of muscle force appropriate for effective interaction with task objects.

    Moves—Pushes, pulls, or drags task objects along a supporting surface.

    Transports—Carries task objects from one place to another while walking, seated in a wheelchair, or using a walker.

    Lifts—Raises or hoists task objects, including lifting an object from one place to another, but without ambulating or moving from one place to another.

    Calibrates—Regulates or grades the force, speed, and extent of movement when interacting with task objects (e.g., not too much or too little).

    Grips—Pinches or grasps task objects with no "grip slips."

- **Energy**—Refers to sustained effort over the course of task performance.

    Endures—Persists and completes the task without obvious evidence of physical fatigue, pausing to rest, or stopping to "catch one's breath."

    Paces—Maintains a consistent and effective rate or tempo of performance throughout the steps of the entire task.

▨ PROCESS SKILLS
—"Skills…used in managing and modifying actions en route to the completion of daily life tasks" (Fisher & Kielhofner, 1995, p. 120).

- **Energy**—Refers to sustained effort over the course of task performance.

    Paces—Maintains a consistent and effective rate or tempo of performance throughout the steps of the entire task.

(Continued)

Appendix B. Performance Skills

(Continued)

Attends—Maintains focused attention throughout the task such that the client is not distracted away from the task by extraneous auditory or visual stimuli.

- **Knowledge**—Refers to the ability to seek and use task-related knowledge.

Chooses—Selects appropriate and necessary tools and materials for the task, including choosing the tools and materials that were specified for use prior to the initiation of the task.

Uses—Uses tools and materials according to their intended purposes and in a reasonable or hygienic fashion, given their intrinsic properties and the availability (or lack of availability) of other objects.

Handles—Supports, stabilizes, and holds tools and materials in an appropriate manner that protects them from damage, falling, or dropping.

Heeds—Uses goal-directed task actions that are focused toward the completion of the specified task (i.e., the outcome originally agreed on or specified by another) without behavior that is driven or guided by environmental cues (i.e., "environmentally cued" behavior).

Inquires—(a) Seeks needed verbal or written information by asking questions or reading directions or labels or (b) asks no unnecessary information questions (e.g., questions related to where materials are located or how a familiar task is performed).

- **Temporal organization**—Pertains to the beginning, logical ordering, continuation, and completion of the steps and action sequences of a task.

Initiates—Starts or begins the next action or step without hesitation.

Continues—Performs actions or action sequences of steps without unnecessary interruption such that once an action sequence is initiated, the individual continues on until the step is completed.

Sequences—Performs steps in an effective or logical order for efficient use of time and energy and with an absence of (a) randomness in the ordering and/or (b) inappropriate repetition ("reordering") of steps.

Terminates—Brings to completion single actions or single steps without perseveration, inappropriate persistence, or premature cessation.

- **Organizing space and objects**—Pertains to skills for organizing task spaces and task objects.

Searches/locates—Looks for and locates tools and materials in a logical manner, including looking beyond the immediate environment (e.g., looking in, behind, on top of).

Gathers—Collects together needed or misplaced tools and materials, including (a) collecting located supplies into the workspace and (b) collecting and replacing materials that have spilled, fallen, or been misplaced.

Organizes—Logically positions or spatially arranges tools and materials in an orderly fashion (a) within a single workspace and (b) among multiple appropriate workspaces to facilitate ease of task performance.

Restores—(a) Puts away tools and materials in appropriate places, (b) restores immediate workspace to original condition (e.g., wiping surfaces clean), (c) closes and seals containers and coverings when indicated, and (d) twists or folds any plastic bags to seal.

Navigates—Modifies the movement pattern of the arm, body, or wheelchair to maneuver around obstacles that are encountered in the course of moving through space such that undesirable contact with obstacles (e.g., knocking over, bumping into) is avoided (includes maneuvering objects held in the hand around obstacles).

- **Adaptation**—Relates to the ability to anticipate, correct for, and benefit by learning from the consequences of errors that arise in the course of task performance.

Notices/responds—Responds appropriately to (a) nonverbal environmental/perceptual cues (i.e., movement, sound, smell, heat, moisture, texture, shape, consistency) that provide feedback with respect to task progression and (b) the spatial arrangement of objects to one another (e.g., aligning objects during stacking). Notices and, when indicated, makes an effective and efficient response.

Accommodates—Modifies his or her actions or the location of objects within the workspace in anticipation of or in response to problems that might arise. The client anticipates or responds to problems effectively by (a) changing the method with which he or she is performing an action sequence, (b) changing the manner in which he or she interacts with or handles tools and materials already in the workspace, and (c) asking for assistance when appropriate or needed.

Adjusts—Changes working environments in anticipation of or in response to problems that might arise. The client anticipates or responds to problems effectively by making some change (a) between working environments by moving to a new workspace or bringing in or removing tools and materials from the present workspace or (b) in an environmental condition (e.g., turning on or off the tap, turning up or down the temperature).

Benefits—Anticipates and prevents undesirable circumstances or problems from recurring or persisting.

- ▨ **COMMUNICATION/INTERACTION SKILLS**—Refer to conveying intentions and needs and coordinating social behavior to act together with people (Forsyth & Kielhofner, 1999; Forsyth, Salamy, Simon, & Kielhofner, 1997; Kielhofner, 2002).

- **Physicality**—Pertains to using the physical body when communicating within an occupation.

Contacts—Makes physical contact with others.

Gazes—Uses eyes to communicate and interact with others.

Gestures—Uses movements of the body to indicate, demonstrate, or add emphasis.

Maneuvers—Moves one's body in relation to others.

Orients—Directs one's body in relation to others and/or occupational forms.

Postures—Assumes physical positions.

- **Information exchange**—Refers to giving and receiving information within an occupation.

Articulates—Produces clear, understandable speech.

Asks—Requests factual or personal information.

Asserts—Directly expresses desires, refusals, and requests.

Engages—Initiates interactions.

Expresses—Displays affect/attitude.

Modulates—Uses volume and inflection in speech.

Shares—Gives out factual or personal information.

Speaks—Makes oneself understood through use of words, phrases, and sentences.

Sustains—Keeps up speech for appropriate duration.

- **Relations**—Relates to maintaining appropriate relationships within an occupation.

Collaborates—Coordinates action with others toward a common end goal.

Conforms—Follows implicit and explicit social norms.

Focuses—Directs conversation and behavior to ongoing social action.

Relates—Assumes a manner of acting that tries to establish a rapport with others.

Respects—Accommodates to other people's reactions and requests.

Note. The Motor and Process Skills sections of this table were compiled from the following sources: Fisher (2001), Fisher and Kielhofner (1995)—updated by Fisher (2001). The Communication/Interaction Skills section of this table was compiled from the following sources: Forsyth and Kielhofner (1999), Forsyth, Salamy, Simon, and Kielhofner (1997), and Kielhofner (2002). From *Occupational therapy practice framework: Domain and process*, by AOTA, 2002, in *American Journal of Occupational Therapy, 56*, 621–622. Reprinted with permission.

Appendix C. Performance Patterns

Patterns of behavior related to daily life activities that are habitual or routine.

▨ **HABITS**—"Automatic behavior that is integrated into more complex patterns that enable people to function on a day-to-day basis" (Neistadt & Crepeau, 1998b, p. 869). Habits can either support or interfere with performance in areas of occupation.

Type of Habit	Examples
• Useful habits	
Habits that support performance in daily life and contribute to life satisfaction.	– Always put car keys in the same place so they can be found easily.
Habits that support ability to follow rhythms of daily life.	– Brush teeth every morning to maintain good oral hygiene.
• Impoverished habits	
Habits that are not established.	– Inconsistently remembering to look both ways before crossing the street.
Habits that need practice to improve.	– Inability to complete all steps of a self-care routine.
• Dominating habits	
Habits that are so demanding they interfere with daily life.	– Repetitive self-stimulation such as type occurring in autism.
	– Use of chemical substances, resulting in addiction.
Habits that satisfy a compulsive need for order.	– Neatly arranging forks on top of each other in silverware drawer.

▨ **ROUTINES**—"Occupations with established sequences" (Christiansen & Baum, 1997, p. 6).

▨ **ROLES**—"A set of behaviors that have some socially agreed upon function and for which there is an accepted code of norms" (Christiansen & Baum, 1997, p. 603).

Note. Information for Habits section of this table adapted from Dunn (2000). From *Occupational therapy practice framework: Domain and process*, by AOTA, 2002, in *American Journal of Occupational Therapy, 56,* 623. Reprinted with permission.

Appendix D. Context or Contexts

Context (including cultural, physical, social, personal, spiritual, temporal, and virtual) refers to a variety of interrelated conditions within and surrounding the client that influence performance.

Context	Definition	Example
Cultural	Customs, beliefs, activity patterns, behavior standards, and expectations accepted by the society of which the individual is a member. Includes political aspects, such as laws that affect access to resources and affirm personal rights. Also includes opportunities for education, employment, and economic support.	• Ethnicity, family, attitude, beliefs, values
Physical	Nonhuman aspects of contexts. Includes the accessibility to and performance within environments having natural terrain, plants, animals, buildings, furniture, objects, tools, or devices.	• Objects, built environment, natural environment, geographic terrain, sensory qualities of environment
Social	Availability and expectations of significant individuals, such as spouse, friends, and caregivers. Also includes larger social groups that are influential in establishing norms, role expectations, and social routines.	• Relationships with individuals, groups, or organizations; relationships with systems (political, economic, institutional)
Personal	"[F]eatures of the individual that are not part of a health condition or health status" (WHO, 2001, p. 17). Personal context includes age, gender, socioeconomic status, and educational status.	• Twenty-five-year-old unemployed man with a high school diploma
Spiritual	The fundamental orientation of a person's life; that which inspires and motivates that individual.	• Essence of the person, greater or higher purpose, meaning, substance
Temporal	"Location of occupational performance in time" (Neistadt & Crepeau, 1998b, p. 292).	• Stages of life, time of day, time of year, duration
Virtual	Environment in which communication occurs by means of airways or computers and an absence of physical contact.	• Realistic simulation of an environment, chat rooms, radio transmissions

Note. Some of the definitions for areas of context or contexts are from the rescinded *Uniform Terminology for Occupational Therapy—Third Edition* (AOTA, 1994b). From *Occupational therapy practice framework: Domain and process*, by AOTA, 2002, in *American Journal of Occupational Therapy, 56,* 623. Reprinted with permission.

Appendix E. Activity Demands

The aspects of an activity, which include the objects, space, social demands, sequencing or timing, required actions, and required underlying body functions and body structure needed to carry out the activity.

Activity Demand Aspects	Definition	Examples
Objects and their properties	The tools, materials, and equipment used in the process of carrying out the activity	• Tools (scissors, dishes, shoes, volleyball) • Materials (paints, milk, lipstick) • Equipment (workbench, stove, basketball hoop) • Inherent properties (heavy, rough, sharp, colorful, loud, bitter tasting)
Space demands (relates to physical context)	The physical environmental requirements of the activity (e.g., size, arrangement, surface, lighting, temperature, noise, humidity, ventilation)	• Large open space outdoors required for a baseball game
Social demands (relates to social and cultural contexts)	The social structure and demands that may be required by the activity	• Rules of game • Expectations of other participants in activity (e.g., sharing of supplies)
Sequence and timing	The process used to carry out the activity (specific steps, sequence, timing requirements)	• Steps—to make tea: gather cup and tea bag, heat water, pour water into cup, etc. • Sequence—heat water before placing tea bag in water • Timing—leave tea bag to steep for 2 minutes
Required actions	The usual skills that would be required by any performer to carry out the activity. Motor, process, and communication interaction skills should each be considered. The performance skills demanded by an activity will be correlated with the demands of the other activity aspects (i.e., objects, space)	• Gripping handlebar • Choosing a dress from closet • Answering a question
Required body functions	"The physiological functions of body systems (including psychological functions)" (WHO, 2001, p. 10) that are required to support the actions used to perform the activity	• Mobility of joints • Level of consciousness
Required body structures	"Anatomical parts of the body such as organs, limbs, and their components [that support body function]" (WHO, 2001, p. 10) that are required to perform the activity	• Number of hands • Number of eyes

From *Occupational therapy practice framework: Domain and process*, by AOTA, 2002, in *American Journal of Occupational Therapy, 56*, 624. Reprinted with permission.

Appendix F. Client Factors

Those factors that reside within the client and that may affect performance in areas of occupation. Client factors include body functions and body structures. Knowledge about body functions and structures is considered when determining which functions and structures are needed to carry out an occupation/activity and how the body functions and structures may be changed as a result of engaging in an occupation/activity. Body functions are "the physiological functions of body systems (including psychological functions)" (WHO, 2001, p. 10). Body structures are "anatomical parts of the body such as organs, limbs and their components [that support body function]" (WHO, 2001, p. 10).

Client Factor	Selected Classifications from ICF and Occupational Therapy Examples
▨ **BODY FUNCTION CATEGORIES**[a]	
Mental functions (affective, cognitive, perceptual)	
• Global mental functions	*Consciousness functions*—level of arousal, level of consciousness. *Orientation functions*—to person, place, time, self, and others. *Sleep*—amount and quality of sleep. *Note:* Sleep and sleep patterns are assessed in relation to how they affect ability to effectively engage in occupations and in daily life activities. *Temperament and personality functions*—conscientiousness, emotional stability, openness to experience. *Note:* These functions are assessed relative to their influence on the ability to engage in occupations and in daily life activities. *Energy and drive functions*—motivation, impulse control, interests, values.
• Specific mental functions	*Attention functions*—sustained attention, divided attention. *Memory functions*—retrospective memory, prospective memory. *Perceptual functions*—visuospatial perception, interpretation of sensory stimuli (tactile, visual, auditory, olfactory, gustatory). *Thought functions*—recognition, categorization, generalization, awareness of reality, logical/coherent thought, appropriate thought content.

(Continued)

Appendix F. Client Factors

(Continued)

Client Factor	Selected Classifications from ICF and Occupational Therapy Examples
	Higher-level cognitive functions—judgment, concept formation, time management, problem solving, decision-making.
	Mental functions of language—able to receive language and express self through spoken and written or sign language. *Note:* This function is assessed relative to its influence on the ability to engage in occupations and in daily life activities.
	Calculation functions—able to add or subtract. *Note:* These functions are assessed relative to their influence on the ability to engage in occupations and in daily life activities (e.g., making change when shopping).
	Mental functions of sequencing complex movement—motor planning.
	Psychomotor functions—appropriate range and regulation of motor response to psychological events.
	Emotional functions—appropriate range and regulation of emotions, self-control.
	Experience of self and time functions—body image, self-concept, self-esteem.
Sensory functions and pain	
• Seeing and related functions	*Seeing functions*—visual acuity, visual field functions.
• Hearing and vestibular functions	*Hearing function*—response to sound. *Note:* This function is assessed in terms of its presence or absence and its affect on engaging in occupations and in daily life activities.
	Vestibular function—balance.
• Additional sensory functions	*Taste function*—ability to discriminate taste.
	Smell function—ability to discriminate smell.
	Proprioceptive function—kinesthesia, joint position sense.
	Touch functions—sensitivity to touch, ability to discriminate.
	Sensory functions related to temperature and other stimuli—sensitivity to temperature, sensitivity to pressure, ability to discriminate temperature and pressure.
• Pain	*Sensations of pain*—dull pain, stabbing pain.
Neuromusculoskeletal and movement-related functions	
• Functions of joints and bones	*Mobility of joint functions*—passive range of motion.
	Stability of joint functions—postural alignment. *Note:* This refers to physiological stability of the joint related to its structural integrity as compared to the motor skill of aligning the body while moving in relation to task objects.
	Mobility of bone functions—frozen scapula, movement of carpal bones.
• Muscle functions	*Muscle power functions*—strength.
	Muscle tone functions—degree of muscle tone (e.g., flaccidity, spasticity).
	Muscle endurance functions—endurance.
• Movement functions	*Motor reflex functions*—stretch reflex, asymmetrical tonic neck reflex.
	Involuntary movement reaction functions—righting reactions, supporting reactions.
	Control of voluntary movement functions—eye–hand coordination, bilateral integration, eye–foot coordination.
	Involuntary movement functions—tremors, tics, motor perseveration.
	Gait pattern functions—walking patterns and impairments, such as asymmetric gait, stiff gait. *Note:* Gait patterns are assessed in relation to how they affect ability to engage in occupations and in daily life activities.
Cardiovascular, hematological, immunological, and respiratory system functions	
• Cardiovascular system function	*Blood pressure functions*—hypertension, hypotension, postural hypotension.
• Hematological and immunological system function	Occupational therapists and occupational therapy assistants have knowledge of these body functions and understand broadly the interaction that occurs between these functions and engagement in occupation to support participation. Some therapists may specialize in evaluating and intervening with a specific function as it is related to supporting performance and engagement in occupations and activities targeted for intervention.

(Continued)

Appendix F. Client Factors

(Continued)

Client Factor	Selected Classifications from ICF and Occupational Therapy Examples
• Respiratory system function	*Respiration functions*—rate, rhythm, and depth.
• Additional functions and sensations of the cardiovascular and respiratory systems	*Exercise tolerance functions*—physical endurance, aerobic capacity, stamina, and fatigability.
Voice and speech functions	
Digestive, metabolic, and endocrine system functions	
• Digestive system functions • Metabolic system and endocrine system functions	Occupational therapists and occupational therapy assistants have knowledge of these body functions and understand broadly the interaction that occurs between these functions and engagement in occupation to support participation. Some therapists may specialize in evaluating and intervening with a specific function as it is related to supporting performance and engagement in occupations and activities targeted for intervention.
Genitourinary and reproductive functions	
• Urinary functions • Genital and reproductive functions	
Skin and related structure functions	
• Skin functions	*Protective functions of the skin*—presence or absence of wounds, cuts, or abrasions. *Repair function of the skin*—wound healing.
• Hair and nail functions	Occupational therapists and occupational therapy assistants have knowledge of these body functions and understand broadly the interaction that occurs between these functions and engagement in occupation to support participation. Some therapists may specialize in evaluating and intervening with a specific function as it is related to supporting performance and engagement in occupations and activities targeted for intervention.

Client Factor	Classifications (Classification are not delineated in the Body Structure section of this table)
■ **BODY STRUCTURE CATEGORIES**[b]	
Structure of the nervous system **The eye, ear, and related structures** **Structures involved in voice and speech** **Structures of the cardiovascular, immunological, and respiratory systems** **Structures related to the digestive system** **Structure related to the genitourinary and reproductive systems** **Structures related to movement** **Skin and related structures**	Occupational therapists and occupational therapy assistants have knowledge of these body functions and understand broadly the interaction that occurs between these functions and engagement in occupation to support participation. Some therapists may specialize in evaluating and intervening with a specific function as it is related to supporting performance and engagement in occupations and activities targeted for intervention.

Note. The reader is strongly encouraged to use *International Classification of Functioning, Disability and Health* (ICF) in collaboration with this table to provide for in-depth information with respect to classification in terms (inclusion and exclusion). From *Occupational therapy practice framework: Domain and process*, by AOTA, 2002, in *American Journal of Occupational Therapy, 56,* 624–626. Reprinted with permission.

[a]Categories and classifications are adapted from the ICF (WHO, 2001). [b]Categories are from the ICF (WHO, 2001).

Appendix G. Occupational Therapy Intervention Approaches

Specific strategies selected to direct the process of intervention that are based on the client's desired outcome, evaluation data, and evidence.

Approach	Focus of Intervention	Examples
Create, promote (health promotion)[a]—an intervention approach that does not assume a disability is present or that any factors would interfere with performance. This approach is designed to provide enriched contextual and activity experiences that will enhance performance for all persons in the natural contexts of life (adapted from Dunn, McClain, Brown, & Youngstrom, 1998, p. 534).	**Performance skills**	• Create a parenting class for first-time parents to teach child development information (performance skill).
	Performance patterns	• Promote handling stress by creating time-use routines with healthy clients (performance pattern).
	Context or contexts	• Create a variety of equipment available at public playgrounds to promote a diversity of sensory play experiences (context).
	Activity demands	• Promote the establishment of sufficient space to allow senior residents to participate in congregate cooking (activity demand).
	Client factors (body functions, body structures)	• Promote increased endurance in school children by having them ride bicycles to school (client factor: body function).
Establish, restore (remediation, restoration)[a]—an intervention approach designed to change client variables to establish a skill or ability that has not yet developed or to restore a skill or ability that has been impaired (adapted from Dunn et al., 1998, p. 533).	**Performance skills**	• Improve coping needed for changing workplace demands by improving assertiveness skills (performance skill).
	Performance patterns	• Establish morning routines needed to arrive at school or work on time (performance pattern).
	Client factors (body functions, body structures)	• Restore mobility needed for play activities (client factor: body function).
Maintain—an intervention approach designed to provide the supports that will allow clients to preserve their performance capabilities that they have regained, that continue to meet their occupational needs, or both. The assumption is that without continued maintenance intervention, performance would decrease, occupational needs would not be met, or both, thereby affecting health and quality of life.	**Performance skills**	• Maintain the ability to organize tools by providing a tool outline painted on a pegboard (performance skill).
	Performance patterns	• Maintain appropriate medication schedule by providing a timer (performance pattern).
	Context or contexts	• Maintain safe and independent access for persons with low vision by providing increased hallway lighting (context).
	Activity demands	• Maintain independent gardening for persons with arthritic hands by providing tools with modified grips (activity demand).
	Client factors (body functions, body structures)	• Maintain proper digestive system functions by developing a dining program (client factor: body function).
		• Maintain upper-extremity muscles necessary for independent wheelchair mobility by developing an after-school–based exercise program (client factor: body structure).
Modify (compensation, adaptation)[a]—an intervention approach directed at "finding ways to revise the current context or activity demands to support performance in the natural setting…[includes] compensatory techniques, including enhancing some features to provide cues, or reducing other features to reduce distractibility" (Dunn et al., 1998, p. 533).	**Context or contexts**	• Modify holiday celebration activities to exclude alcohol to support sobriety (context).
	Activity demands	• Modify office equipment (e.g. chair, computer station) to support individual employee body function and performance skill abilities (activity demand).
	Performance patterns	• Modify daily routines to provide consistency and predictability to support individual's cognitive ability (performance pattern).
Prevent (disability prevention)[a]—an intervention approach designed to address clients with or without a disability who are at risk for occupational performance problems. This approach is designed to prevent the occurrence or evolution of barriers to performance in context. Interventions may be directed at client, context, or activity variables (adapted from Dunn et al., 1998, p. 534).	**Performance skills**	• Prevent poor posture when sitting for prolonged periods by providing a chair with proper back support (performance skill).
	Performance patterns	• Prevent the use of chemical substances by introducing self-initiated strategies to assist in remaining drug free (performance pattern).
	Context or contexts	• Prevent social isolation by suggesting participation in after-work group activities (context).
	Activity demands	• Prevent back injury by providing instruction in proper lifting techniques (activity demand).
	Client factors (body functions, body structures)	• Prevent increased blood pressure during homemaking activities by learning to monitor blood pressure in a cardiac exercise program (client factor: body function).
		• Prevent repetitive stress injury by suggesting that a wrist support splint be worn when typing (client factor: body structure).

[a]Parallel language used in Moyers (1999, p. 274). From *Occupational therapy practice framework: Domain and process*, by AOTA, 2002, in *American Journal of Occupational Therapy, 56*, 627. Reprinted with permission.

Appendix H. Types of Occupational Therapy Interventions

THERAPEUTIC USE OF SELF—A practitioner's planned use of his or her personality, insights, perceptions, and judgments as part of the therapeutic process (adapted from Punwar & Peloquin, 2000, p. 285).

THERAPEUTIC USE OF OCCUPATIONS AND ACTIVITIES[a]—Occupations and activities selected for specific clients that meet therapeutic goals. To use occupations/activities therapeutically, context or contexts, activity demands, and client factors all should be considered in relation to the client's therapeutic goals.

Occupation-based activity	*Purpose:* Allows clients to engage in actual occupations that are part of their own context and that match their goals.
	Examples:
	• Play on playground equipment during recess
	• Purchase own groceries and prepare a meal
	• Adapt the assembly line to achieve greater safety
	• Put on clothes without assistance
Purposeful activity	*Purpose:* Allows the client to engage in goal-directed behaviors or activities within a therapeutically designed context that lead to an occupation or occupations.
	Examples:
	• Practice vegetable slicing
	• Practice drawing a straight line
	• Practice safe ways to get in and out of a bathtub equipped with grab bars
	• Role-play to learn ways to manage anger
Preparatory methods	*Purpose:* Prepares the client for occupational performance. Used in preparation for purposeful and occupation-based activities.
	Examples:
	• Sensory input to promote optimum response
	• Physical agent modalities
	• Orthotics/splinting (design, fabrication, application)
	• Exercise

CONSULTATION PROCESS—A type of intervention in which practitioners use their knowledge and expertise to collaborate with the client. The collaborative process involves identifying the problem, creating possible solutions, trying solutions, and altering them as necessary for greater effectiveness. When providing consultation, the practitioner is not directly responsible for the outcome of the intervention (Dunn, 2000, p. 113).

EDUCATION PROCESS—An intervention process that involves the imparting of knowledge and information about occupation and activity and that does not result in the actual performance of the occupation/activity.

From *Occupational therapy practice framework: Domain and process*, by AOTA, 2002, in *American Journal of Occupational Therapy, 56*, 628. Reprinted with permission.
[a]Information adapted from Pedretti and Early (2001).

Appendix I. Types of Occupational Therapy Outcomes

The examples listed specify how the broad outcome of engagement in occupation may be operationalized. The examples are not intended to be all-inclusive.

Outcome	Description
Occupational performance	The ability to carry out activities of daily life (areas of occupation). Occupational performance can be addressed in two different ways:
	• Improvement—used when a performance deficit is present, often as a result of an injury or disease process. This approach results in increased independence and function in ADL, IADL, education, work, play, leisure, or social participation.
	• Enhancement—used when a performance deficit is not currently present. This approach results in the development of performance skills and performance patterns that augment performance or prevent potential problems from developing in daily life occupations.
Client satisfaction	The client's affective response to his or her perceptions of the process and benefits of receiving occupational therapy services (adapted from Maciejewski, Kawiecki, & Rockwood, 1997).
Role competence	The ability to effectively meet the demand of roles in which the client engages.
Adaptation	"A change a person makes in his or her response approach when that person encounters an occupational challenge. This change is implemented when the individual's customary response approaches are found inadequate for producing some degree of mastery over the challenge" (Christiansen & Baum, 1997, p. 591).
Health and wellness	*Health*—"A complete state of physical, mental, and social well-being and not just the absence of disease or infirmity" (WHO, 1947, p. 29).
	Wellness—The condition of being in good health, including the appreciation and the enjoyment of health. Wellness is more than a lack of disease symptoms; it is a state of mental and physical balance and fitness (adapted from *Taber's Cyclopedic Medical Dictionary*, 1997, p. 2110).
Prevention	Promoting a healthy lifestyle at the individual, group, organizational, community (societal), and governmental or policy level (adapted from Brownson & Scaffa, 2001).
Quality of life	A person's dynamic appraisal of his or her life satisfactions (perceptions of progress toward one's goals), self-concept (the composite of beliefs and feelings about oneself), health and functioning (including health status, self-care capabilities, role competence), and socioeconomic factors (e.g., vocation, education, income) (adapted from Radomski, 1995; Zhan, 1992).

Note. ADL = activities of daily living; IADL = instrumental activities of daily living. From *Occupational therapy practice framework: Domain and process*, by AOTA, 2002, in *American Journal of Occupational Therapy, 56*, 628. Reprinted with permission.

Appendix J.

CLIENT PROFILE AND TASK ANALYSIS FORM

CLIENT PROFILE

Name:

Occupational history:

Patterns of daily living (see also performance patterns):

Interests, values, and needs:

TASK ANALYSIS

Task:

ACTIVITY DEMANDS

Objects used:

Space demands:

Social demands:

Sequence and timing:

Required actions:
1.
2.
3.
4.
5.
6.
7.
8.
9.
10.

AREAS OF OCCUPATION

Check the area or areas that apply. ☑	*Relevance and meaning for client:*
Activities of daily living (ADL) ☐	_____
Instrumental ADL ☐	_____
Education ☐	_____
Work ☐	_____
Play ☐	_____
Leisure ☐	_____
Social participation ☐	_____

PERFORMANCE PATTERNS

Habits:

Routines:

Roles:

Continued

Appendix J. *(Continued)*

PERFORMANCE SKILLS

Qualifiers: 0 (no impairment), 1 (mild impairment), 2 (moderate impairment), 3 (severe impairment),
4 (complete impairment), 8 (not specified), 9 (not applicable)

Motor Skills		*Qualifier*	*Process Skills*		*Qualifier*
Posture:	Stabilizes	☐	Energy:	Paces	☐
	Aligns	☐		Attends	☐
	Positions	☐	Knowledge:	Chooses	☐
Mobility:	Walks	☐		Uses	☐
	Reaches	☐		Handles	☐
	Bends	☐		Heeds	☐
Coordination:	Coordinates	☐		Inquires	☐
	Manipulates	☐	Temporal		
	Flows	☐	organization:	Initiates	☐
Strength and effort:	Moves	☐		Continues	☐
	Transports	☐		Sequences	☐
	Lifts	☐		Terminates	☐
	Calibrates	☐	Organization of		
	Grips	☐	space and objects:	Searches or locates	☐
Energy:	Endures	☐		Gathers	☐
	Paces	☐		Organizes	☐
Comments:				Restores	☐
				Navigates	☐
			Adaptation:	Notices or responds	☐
				Accommodates	☐
				Adjusts	☐
				Benefits	☐
			Comments:		

Communication and Interaction Skills

		Qualifier			*Qualifier*
Posture:	Contacts	☐	Information	Articulates	☐
	Gazes	☐	exchange:	Asserts	☐
	Gestures	☐		Engages	☐
	Maneuvers	☐		Expresses	☐
	Orients	☐		Modulates	☐
	Postures	☐		Shares	☐
Relations:	Collaborates	☐		Speaks	☐
	Conforms	☐		Sustains	☐
	Focuses	☐	*Comments:*		
	Relates	☐			
	Respects	☐			

Continued

Appendix J. *(Continued)*

ACTIVITY DEMANDS AND CLIENT FACTORS

Activity demand qualifiers
Level of challenge required to perform:
1 (mild challenge), 2 (moderate challenge),
3 (maximum challenge), 9 (not applicable)

Client factor qualifiers
Level of client impairment: 0 (no impairment), 1 (mild impairment), 2 (moderate impairment), 3 (severe impairment), 4 (complete impairment), 8 (not specified), 9 (not applicable)

Level of Demand
Comments and qualifier:

Level of Impairment
Qualifier and comments:

Body Functions

Mental functions: Global

☐ Consciousness functions ☐
☐ Orientation functions ☐
☐ Sleep ☐
☐ Temperament and ☐
  personality functions
☐ Energy and drive functions ☐

Mental functions: Specific

☐ Attention functions ☐
☐ Memory functions ☐
☐ Perceptual functions ☐
☐ Thought functions ☐
☐ Higher-level cognitive functions ☐
☐ Mental functions of language ☐
☐ Calculation functions ☐
☐ Mental functions of sequencing ☐
  complex movement
☐ Psychomotor functions ☐
☐ Emotional functions ☐
☐ Experience of self and time ☐
  functions

Sensory functions and pain

☐ Seeing functions ☐
☐ Hearing functions ☐
☐ Vestibular functions ☐
☐ Taste functions ☐
☐ Smell functions ☐
☐ Proprioceptive functions ☐
☐ Touch functions ☐
☐ Sensory functions related to ☐
  temperature and other stimuli
☐ Sensations of pain ☐

Neuromusculoskeletal and movement-related functions

☐ Mobility of joint functions ☐
☐ Stability of joint functions ☐
☐ Mobility of bone functions ☐
☐ Muscle power functions ☐
☐ Muscle tone functions ☐
☐ Muscle endurance functions ☐
☐ Motor reflex functions ☐
☐ Involuntary movement reaction ☐
  functions
☐ Control of voluntary movement ☐
  functions
☐ Involuntary movement ☐
  functions
☐ Gait pattern functions ☐

Continued

ACTIVITY DEMANDS AND CLIENT FACTORS

Cardiovascular and respiratory systems

_____	☐	Blood pressure functions	☐ _____
_____	☐	Respiration functions	☐ _____
_____	☐	Exercise tolerance functions	☐ _____

Skin and related structure functions

_____	☐	Protective functions of the skin	☐ _____
_____	☐	Repair functions of the skin	☐ _____

Body Structures

_____ ☐ Structure of the nervous system ☐ _____

_____ ☐ Eye, ear, and related structures ☐ _____

_____ ☐ Structures involved in voice ☐ _____
          and speech

_____ ☐ Structures of the cardiovascular, ☐ _____
          immunological, and
          respiratory systems
          Additional Comments:

_____ ☐ Structures related to the ☐ _____
          digestive system
          Additional Comments:

_____ ☐ Structures related to the ☐ _____
          genitourinary and
          reproductive system
          Additional Comments:

_____ ☐ Structures related to ☐ _____
          movement
          Additional Comments:

_____ ☐ Skin and related ☐ _____
          structures
          Additional Comments:

CONTEXTS

External to the Client

Cultural context (e.g., laws, resources, opportunities):

Physical context:

Social context:

Temporal context (e.g., time of day, year):

Virtual context:

Internal to the Client

Personal context:

Spiritual context:

Cultural context (e.g., customs, values, beliefs):

Temporal context (e.g., age, stage of life):

Appendix K. Writing Effective Client Goals and Objectives

As part of the evaluation process, occupational therapists work in partnership with clients and their families, caregivers, and other stakeholders to develop priorities, goals, and objectives in dimensions thought to affect engagement in occupations and participation in contexts. These priorities, goals, and objectives guide the transition to the intervention process, and they form the basis for the therapeutic strategies the practitioner designs and implements.

Client priorities reflect the values, beliefs, and needs associated with the client's activity limitations and participation restrictions. Priorities are identified in areas of occupations, roles, and responsibilities that are meaningful to the client. Client priorities provide the foundation on which goals and objectives are established.

Goals define expected outcomes in engagement in occupations, participation in contexts, role competency, quality of life, adaptation, lifestyles, health, and wellness. Goals are long term in nature. They must be specific, objective rather than subjective, and measurable and clearly identify the individual or entity that is to achieve the desired outcome.

Objectives are short term in nature and relate to or are sequenced steps toward long-term goals. Objectives identify the dimensions in which change is expected. For example, specific performance skills and patterns or client factors may need to be developed, restored, or maintained as a step toward accomplishing the goal. Furthermore, objectives may address activity demands that must be met and performance contexts that must be modified or augmented to enable the client to compensate or adapt. Objectives may also relate to steps that will be taken to promote health or prevent disability. Just like goals, objectives must be specific, objective rather than subjective, and measurable and clearly identify the individual or entity that is to achieve the desired outcome. A format for writing goals and objectives is provided in Table K.1, and Figure K.1 illustrates the process of writing goals and objectives using the example of Bobbie from the case study in chapter 7.

To develop effective goals and objectives, occupational therapy practitioners use task analysis to analyze the dynamic interaction among a client, a selected task, and specific contexts. Task analysis is useful in breaking down client goals into objectives and objectives into smaller, doable, and measurable units of activity that are sequenced to facilitate success but provoke challenge.

Task analysis also helps practitioners identify *resources,* which are the assets available to help clients works toward goal achievement. Resources may be tangible, such as physical and financial assets, or intangible, such as social support and political will. Skilled and knowledgeable practitioners and the evaluation and intervention services they provide can be considered to be resources available to clients.

Table K.1. Format for Writing Client Goals and Objectives.

Long-Term Goal	Short-Term Objectives
1.	1a.
	1b.
2.	2a.
	2b.
3.	3a.
	3b.
4.	4a.
	4b.

Effective goals and objectives contain the following elements:

Who → **will do** → **what** → **from what level** → **to what level** → **by when** → **using what resources**

Goal: Bobbie will ride his tricycle through an obstacle course with improved speed and agility as demonstrated by ease of performance and increased participation within 6 weeks with daily opportunity to practice.

Element	Description	Example
Who	Identifies the client as the person, group, or population invested in achieving the goal	Bobbie
Will do	Describes the desired direction of the change—e.g., increase, decrease	Will improve
What	Identifies the area of occupation, performance skill or pattern, or client function targeted for intervention	Ride a tricycle through an obstacle course
From what level	Provide brief description of element	Current performance
To what level	Provide brief description of element	With speed and agility With ease of performance With increased participation
By when	Provide brief description of element	Within 6 weeks
Using what resources	Provide brief description of element	Daily opportunity to practice

Objective: Bobbie will ride his tricycle up and down slight inclines with confidence within 2 weeks with daily opportunity to practice.

Element	Description	Example
Who	Identifies the client as the person, group, or population invested in achieving the goal	Bobbie
Will do	Describes the desired direction of the change—e.g., increase, decrease	Will improve
What	Identifies the area of occupation, performance skill or pattern, or client function targeted for intervention	Ride a tricycle
From what level	Provide brief description of element	Current performance
To what level	Provide brief description of element	Up and down slight inclines with confidence
By when	Provide brief description of element	Within 2 weeks
Using what resources	Provide brief description of element	Daily opportunity to practice

Figure K.1. Elements of effective client goals and objectives and example goals and objectives for Bobbie, a 5-year-old boy (see full case study in chapter 7).

Appendix L. AOTA Position Paper: Purposeful Activity

The American Occupational Therapy Association, Inc., submits this paper to clarify the use of the term purposeful activity, a central focus of occupational therapy throughout its history. People engage in purposeful activity as part of their daily life routines, in the context of occupational performance (Resolution C, 1979). Occupation refers to active participation in self-maintenance, work, leisure, and play. Purposeful activity refers to goal-directed behaviors or tasks that comprise occupations. An activity is purposeful if the individual is an active, voluntary participant and if the activity is directed toward a goal that the individual considers meaningful (Evans, 1987; Gilfoyle, 1984; Mosey, 1986; Nelson, 1988). The purposefulness of an activity lies with the individual performing the activity and with the context in which it is done (Henderson et al., 1991). The meaning of an activity is unique to each person, influenced by his or her life experiences (Mosey, 1986; Pedretti, 1982), life roles, interests, age, and cultural background, as well as the situational context in which the activity occurs. Occupational therapy practitioners[1] are committed to the use of purposeful activity to evaluate, facilitate, restore, or maintain individuals' abilities to function in their daily occupations.

Occupational therapists use activities to evaluate an individual's capacities to meet the functional demands of his or her environment and daily life. Based on an evaluation, the occupational therapy practitioner, in collaboration with the individual, designs activity experiences that offer the individual opportunities for effective action. Purposeful activities assist and build upon the individual's abilities and lead to achievement of personal functional goals.

Purposeful activity provides opportunities for persons to achieve mastery of their environment, and successful performance promotes feelings of personal competence (Fidler & Fidler, 1978). A person who is involved in purposeful activity directs attention to the goal rather than to the processes required for achievement of the goal. Engagement in purposeful activity within the context of interpersonal, cultural, physical, and other environmental conditions requires and elicits coordination among the individual's sensory motor, cognitive, and psychosocial systems. Purposeful activity may involve the independent use of complex cognitive processes, such as premeditation, reflection, planning, and use of symbolic cues. Conversely, it may involve less complex processes and take place in an environment of external structure, support, and supervision (Allen, 1987; Henderson et al., 1991). Engagement in purposeful activity provides direct and objective feedback of performance both to the occupational therapy practitioner and the individual.

The therapeutic purposes for which purposeful activity is used include mastery of a new skill, restoration of a deficient ability, compensation for functional disability, health maintenance, or prevention of dysfunction. To use purposeful activity therapeutically, an occupational practitioner analyzes the activity from several perspectives. First, the activity is examined to identify its component parts to determine which skills and abilities are necessary to complete the task. Second, it is examined in terms of the context in which it will be performed. Third, the practitioner considers the person's age, occupational roles, cultural background, gender, interests, and preferences that may influence the meaningfulness of the activity for the individual. All this information is considered together to assist the occupational therapy practitioner in synthesizing (i.e., adapting, grading, and combining) activities for therapeutic purposes for a particular individual.

Purposeful activities cannot be prescribed based on analysis of their inherent characteristics

---

[1] *Occupational therapy practitioners*—refers to both registered occupational therapists and certified occupational therapy assistants.

198

alone; rather, by definition, prescription of purposeful activity is individual-specific. An occupational therapy practitioner grades or adapts a chosen activity for an individual to promote successful performance or elicit a particular response. Grading activities challenges the patient's abilities by progressively changing the process, tools, materials, or environment of a given activity to gradually increase or decrease performance demands. These incremental modifications are made in response to the individual's dynamic changes and provide opportunities for gradual development of skill and related therapeutic benefits. The grading of activities is accomplished by modifying the sequence, duration, or procedures of the task; the individual's position; the position of the tools and materials; the size, shape, weight, or texture of the materials; the nature and degree of interpersonal contact; the extent of physical handling by the occupational therapy practitioner during performance; or the environment in which the activity is attempted. Supportive or assistive devices or techniques may be used to enhance the effectiveness of an activity or to facilitate performance (Henderson et al., 1991; Pedretti & Pasquinelli, 1990). Such techniques or devices are considered facilitative or preparatory to performance of purposeful activity and engagement in occupations.

If the therapy goal is to enhance a performance component so that an individual can engage in an occupational performance area, the selected activity and environmental conditions are manipulated to present graded challenges to the specific skills required. When an individual's successful completion of a task is a priority, occupational therapy practitioners adapt the task and the environment to facilitate performance. Adaptation is a process that changes an aspect of the activity or the environment to enable successful performance and accomplish a particular therapeutic goal. Adaptation of a task may require the use of assistive devices and techniques or grading strategies.

Occupational therapy education provides the necessary background for using activities as therapeutic modalities by instructing the student about behavioral and biological sciences related to the use and meaning of activity, about the nature of purposeful activity, about the process of activity analysis and synthesis, and about the application of activity to therapeutic problems within occupational therapy frames of reference.

In summary, purposeful occurs within the context of work, self-care, play, and leisure activities and is used therapeutically to evaluate, facilitate, restore, or maintain individual's abilities to function competently within their daily occupations. The occupational therapy practitioner's commitment to those he or she serves is to guide them in the use of purposeful activities so as to empower them to enhance the quality of their being in the daily reality where they live as parents, children, students, homemakers, workers, or retirees (Reilly, 1966).

References

Allen, C. K. (1987). Activity: Occupational therapy's treatment method. *American Journal of Occupational Therapy, 41,* 563–575.

Evans, A. K. (1987). Nationally Speaking: Definition of occupation as the core concept of occupational therapy. *American Journal of Occupational Therapy, 41,* 627–628.

Fidler, G. S., & Fidler, J. W. (1978). Doing and becoming: Purposeful action and self actualization. *American Journal of Occupational Therapy, 32,* 305–310.

Gilfoyle, E. (1984). Eleanor Clarke Slagle Lectureship, 1984: Transformation of a profession. *American Journal of Occupational Therapy, 38,* 575–584.

Henderson, A., Cermak, S., Coster, W., Murray, E., Trombly, C., & Tickle-Degnen, L. (1991). The Issue Is—Occupational science is multidimensional. *American Journal of Occupational Therapy, 45,* 370–372.

Mosey, A. C. (1986). *Psychosocial components of occupational therapy.* New York: Raven Press.

Nelson, D. L. (1988). Occupation: Form and performance. *American Journal of Occupational Therapy, 42,* 633–641.

Appendix L. AOTA Position Paper: Purposeful Activity

(Continued)

Pedretti, L. W. (1982). The compatibility of current treatment methods in physical disabilities with the philosophical base of occupational therapy. Presentation at the American Occupational Therapy Association Annual Conference, Philadelphia, PA, May 1982.

Pedretti, L. W., & Pasquinelli, S. (1990). A frame of reference for occupational therapy in physical dysfunction. In L.W. Pedretti & B. Zoltan (Eds.), *Occupational therapy practice skills for physical dysfunction* (pp. 1–17). St. Louis, MO: Mosby.

Reilly, M. (1966). The challenge of the future to an occupational therapist. *American Journal of Occupational Therapy, 20,* 221–225.

Resolution C, 531–79. The philosophical base of occupational therapy. *American Journal of Occupational Therapy, 33,* 785.

Authors
Jim Hinojosa, PhD, OTR, FAOTA
Joyce Sabari, PhD, OTR
Lorraine Pedretti, MS, OTR
With contributions from
Mark S. Rosenfeld, PhD, OTR
Catherine Trombly, ScD, OTR/L, FAOTA
For Commission on Practice
Jim Hinojosa, PhD, OTR, FAOTA, Chairperson

Approved by the Representative Assembly April 1983
Revised and approved by the Representative Assembly June 1993

Previously published and copyrighted in 1993 by the American Occupational Therapy
Association in the *American Journal of Occupational Therapy, 47,* 1081–1082.

Index

Note: References in *italics* refer to figures.
References in **bold** refer to tables.

About the Authors

Diane E. Watson PhD, MBA, BScOT

Diane Watson has been involved in clinical practice, teaching, and research in occupational therapy in Canada and the United States for 20 years. She is currently assistant director of the Institute of Health Services and Policy Research (IHSPR) in Vancouver. IHSPR is one of 13 institutes that form the Canadian Institutes of Health Research, Canada's premier research funding agency.

Sylvia A. Wilson, MSc, OT

Sylvia Wilson has been involved in clinical practice, teaching, medical–legal private practice, and community development in occupational therapy in Canada and the United States for 30 years. She has been qualified as an expert witness by the Court of Queen's Bench, Alberta, in her role in cost of future care. She is currently centre coordinator for the Centre for Health Promotion Studies at the University of Alberta in Edmonton. The centre was created in 1995 in response to a growing demand for new knowledge and skills in health promotion and population health in a rapidly changing health system. The centre's mandates include graduate education, research, and community service.